Salt and Pepper

Salt and Pepper

You are the Salt of the Earth

Lyle Olmstead

PW Pleasant Word™
A Division of WinePress Group™

Pleasant Word (a division of WinePress Publishing, PO Box 428, Enumclaw, WA 98022) functions only as book publisher. As such, the ultimate design, content, editorial accuracy, and views expressed or implied in this work are those of the author.

ISBN 13: 978-1-4141-1455-2
ISBN 10: 1-4141-1455-9
Library of Congress Catalog Card Number: 2009904121

Contents

Section Two: Family Life

Section Three: Community Life

Section Four: The Modern Age

Section Five: Christianity

Preface

SALT AND PEPPER is a series of articles that are observations on everyday life. These articles have been written over many years. They are intended to cause the reader to think about how his or her life is somewhat similar to the lives of others, both now and in the past.

We humans are created to have personalities that are very different from each other, yet we are similar in many ways. During my observations of the human race from different positions on the globe—be it in China, Pakistan, Australia, Costa Rica, England, or Wales—I saw that people respond to circumstances according to their culture, and yet we all tend to observe life from a similar viewpoint. Yes, our cultural differences are ever present, but two different human beings, given similar situations and opportunities, will respond with sensitivity common to all beings.

To this end I have written down these articles. My hope is that you will enjoy these observations, laugh with some, and cry from reading others. As you read these writings, may you respond in your own particular manner.

Section One

Back in the Day

Washing

TODAY IS SATURDAY. What is so different about that? Each week has a Saturday. Usually on Saturday my wife does part of the week's washing. Today she is doing the whole week's washing in one day. Why? She has been saving the dirty clothes all week to wash them all at one time. Why? Because we are going on vacation, and she wants to have as many of the clothes clean as possible. This is her logic. Men usually would do the same, except we wouldn't be saving up laundry to get it clean for a vacation; we would just allow a couple of weeks' washings to accumulate before we did anything about it. As long as a man has a clean shirt, socks, and underclothes to wear, he is satisfied.

Women and men have it easy when they do the washing today. Gather the clothes from the hamper, place them in the washing machine, and it does the rest. When they are washed, you place them in the dryer or on the clothesline, and "Zippo," one has clean clothes to wear.

Not so with my mother or grandmother. First they had to heat the water, then get the scrub board, find the washtub, and after getting the lie soap, bend over the washtub to scrub the clothes. As if this was not enough, they then had to have another tub to rinse the soap out of the clothes. After that, they carried the clothes to the clothesline and hung them up with clothespins to be dried by the wind. In winter weather, the clothes would freeze. So the person washing the clothes would have to bring the frozen clothes into the house and find some place near the stove to thaw them out and see if they would dry. If the house had a basement or empty room, usually these frozen clothes would be hung in there until dry.

It is little wonder that the early settlers of our nation wore their clothes without washing them in the wintertime. Perfume was used quite often to cover the body odors, or the neighbor in church or a meeting had to sit as far away from the smelly person as possible. Usually the entire crowd smelled the same, so no one was offended.

Until the middle of the last century, most poor or middle class persons had a bath once a week instead of the daily shower now prescribed. Water was difficult to come by, and after pumping it from the well, it was used sparingly.

With the advent of modern indoor plumbing, which we take for granted, the excessive use of water came into play. Even as I sit here writing this article, my wife is running the washer and dryer. In a couple of hours our clothes will be washed and dried for another week. We shall board the airplane with clean clothes to last us for seven days. How? Because we have the modern convenience of indoor plumbing, a washing machine, and a dryer.

The modern conveniences we have cause us to forget how fortunate we are in the Western world. Females in the third world are still using the most basic methods for washing of the body and clothes. To do laundry, first they must find the wood to build a fire. They then carry the water for miles to heat it and wash the clothes by pounding them on rocks and then laying them out on the ground or hanging them from a fence or tree to dry. I often wondered, when living in these countries, how the women were ever able to get their clothes as clean as they did.

I am amazed by the fact that so many people die young or of illnesses in the countries outside of the Western world. With the lack of sanitary necessities, germs thrive and, only the strong survive. The weak die at birth or very early in life.

In the Western world we keep even the sickliest child alive. I am an example of that. In the first eighteen months of my life I contracted scarlet fever and had a relapse. The doctor came to my grandmother's home each day to take care of me. Because of his efforts and those of my grandmother and mother, I have lived for eighty-six years. The "strep bug" that gave me the scarlet fever, however, has lived in my body all these years. And every so often it comes back to let me know that it is lurking just around the corner.

Was it because of the poor sanitary conditions in which I was being reared at that time that I became ill? Or did the "strep bug" just happen to catch me in a weak moment of my young life? Who knows; perhaps it was a combination. Fortunately, the medical doctor who took care of me had many years of experience with fever treatment. He had been a medical missionary in India prior to settling in the city where my grandmother was residing and I was born.

Perhaps this article should have had a different title. What would you have named it?

Country Living

HAVE YOU EVER gone to an outhouse on a cold winter day? How about on a hot summer day? This is my memory of country living. In the wintertime, you would wait until the very last minute and then thrust on warm clothes and rush down the path to the toilet. In the summertime, there were flies and other insects coming up to bite your bottom once you were seated. And if all this was not enough, the toilet paper was the old issue of a mail-order catalog.

This style of country living is in the past for a large portion of our population. In areas outside of the Western world, the situation described above is still common, and even in some portions of the Western world this is still the norm. But really, unless one lives in a back section of our nation today, the present generation cannot comprehend country living as the folks of my generation did. There are areas in the mountains of the nation where these conditions still exist, but for the majority of our population, rural poverty is hard to imagine. So let me give you more of a glimpse of what it was like...

In my early life we lived with primitive facilities most of the time. We pumped the water for drinking and washing from a well outside our home, carried the water in, heated it over the kitchen stove, placed it in the family laundry tub, and then carried the used water outside to dump it from the family washing—both clothes and personal. At least we were not in danger of certain waterborne diseases, because after the health officials learned how disease was carried, the outhouse was placed far away from the fresh water source.

The facilities that were furnished to our family as a portion of the salary my minister father received were primitive living at its best. The old parsonage was very cold in the winter, and hot and humid in the summer. Often in the wintertime I would awaken with frost on the walls of my bedroom. In the summer I would sleep on the porch because the upstairs bedroom was impossibly hot.

My mother, who had to cook meals three times a day for a family of seven, had to work over a cookstove that was fired with coal in the winter and summer; she also had a kerosene stove with three burners.

Country living is a memory I am pleased to forget…

Clothing was very simple. We had one pair of shoes, resoled as often as possible by the father in the family; a pair of jeans; one shirt, worn again and again; and underwear of the long johns type in the winter and briefs in the summer. Undershirts were not a part of our clothing; they cost too much. Winter clothes were passed down from male child to male child, and it was the same for the female children. I am sure we must have smelled of the sweat and other odors the human body takes on.

Until my father was moved to the city or a small town, the above accommodations were the norm. When he was moved to a city or small town, the conditions changed for the better, at least as far as bathing and toilet facilities were concerned. In those times we had indoor plumbing, and the days of carrying water in from the pump to the kitchen stove were over.

In country living we always had some food that my father raised on a half acre of garden in a plot of ground located adjacent to the parsonage. He also kept a cow and chickens, and once a year he would purchase a newborn pig to raise and butcher. In addition, each fall our parents would can all the food they could to feed the five hungry mouths until the next spring, when the cycle would begin all over again. Without all this food help we would have had a difficult time getting enough to eat.

On a positive note, the upside of country living was the fresh, clean air we had to breathe...but still, country living is a memory I am glad to forget.

The Day Before

THE SUSPENSE IS killing me" is what some people say when they have to wait for a long period of time. It reminds me of waiting for a memorial service to begin. We all want it to be over, but we also do not want to neglect the memory of the deceased. Have you ever been in that situation?

When I was a child, it seemed as if Christmas Day would never arrive. You know what I mean. In your head you pictured all the things you had asked Santa to bring you. ADHD had nothing to do with Christmas Eve, but children were jumping all over the place. Mother and Father were attempting to get the children into bed so they could deliver the presents under the tree. Sometimes it was a game of hide-and-seek—the children would attempt to see from behind the curtains what Dad and Mom were placing under the tree for each child. Usually, this all took place after a Christmas Eve service in the local church.

The Depression years were tough, especially as far as the giving of presents. Mom and Dad were having a difficult time feeding the family, and now the extra burden of gift giving for Christmas loomed upon the stage of life. Really, any extra expense was difficult to handle.

Salt and Pepper

The day before Thanksgiving was especially trying for us kids. We knew we usually traveled to Grandma's house, but with money in short supply, we did not know if our parents would decide not to drive that distance. The distance was not really that far; at the most it was fifty or sixty miles from the middle of the state where we lived to the western side where she lived.

Our parents did decide to drive to Grandpa and Grandma's house. Into the Model A Ford we five children would assemble ourselves, the eldest son on the outside window, the eldest daughter on the opposite side of the car, and the three little ones in the middle. This would make it possible for a good scrap to take place. Each child would be juggling to get closer to an outside window. We children actually plotted out the strategy for window conquest the day before we left. And I'm sure our parents knew what progress was being made in the Model A's rear seat on the trip.

The waiting period before we left was really the tough time. We were almost bursting with excitement! We could taste the fried chicken, mashed potatoes, sweet carrots, string beans, and corn. And the final course would be ice cream; that is, if Grandma could afford it. If not, there would be pumpkin and apple pie with whipped cream. No wonder we had a difficult time going to sleep the night before the trip! With all the food fairies dancing in our heads, how did our parents expect us children to go to sleep?

We had the same problem the night before Christmas. After all, when the day before Christmas came and the night before programs were bouncing around their children's heads, how did parents expect anything other than very excited children, with sleep way off in the distant corner of their brains?

Now that I have gone through experiences like this myself, I realize that parents wear out long before their children do. Dads and moms are ready to retire just as the children are getting their second wind. The parents are pooped; the kids are all set for running around the remainder of the evening.

The Day Before

As a parent, I often wished I could have only half of the energy my children had the night before any big event, or half the energy I had when I was a child, for that matter.

The Country Store

HAVE YOU EVER purchased items from a country store? Do you remember the country store where you lived, or did you live in a large city?

When I spent a month in New York City, I was surprised to see many small grocery stores and stores that specialized in a particular group of items or in items for a particular group of people. They might be selling foods from India, Korea, China, and Poland—everything except what we consider to be well-known foods.

Let me tell you about the country store I remember as a child. The location for the store I remember was a spot in the gravel highway named Cohocatah Center. This was the name of a Native American group that had originally been living there until the white man drove him out. The main attractions in that area were the store, the gas station, Grange Hall, and the local Roman Catholic Church.

The country store was a long, wooden structure with a brick front that was built in the early 1900s. There was an awning that could be rolled down when the sun was hot or to keep the rain off you as you entered the building. Large, glass windows ran across the front of the building, and samples displayed inside were of the merchandise for sale.

Inside the store, shelves running the length of the interior of the building covered the walls. At the rear of the store was a large potbellied stove with chairs arranged around it in an irregular fashion. Usually there was a spittoon located nearby to accommodate those who chewed tobacco. Also in the rear of the store, there was a large freezer, which in the early days was stocked with large blocks of ice to keep meats and other perishable foods from spoiling. In later years, the freezer was mechanized to be cooled with refrigeration.

Goods for sale included everything from long underwear to plow points. (The stores today that are most like the country store, except on a much larger scale, are Wal-Mart or Target). If the storekeeper did not have the item you wanted to purchase, he had a catalog from which you could order.

The storekeeper and his wife were on duty from morning until evening. He was a tall, plump fellow, and his wife was short and well endowed. He was a nonbeliever, and his wife attended the church where my father was the pastor. Their home was on the lot adjoining the store. When I knew them as a child, they must have been in their fifties.

The store served two purposes: 1) It provided a place for people in the area to purchase products they needed without having to drive to larger towns ten to twelve miles away. 2) It was the place where local gossip was shared.

In the wintertime the men gathered around the potbellied stove to tell stories and swap gossip. Here they could smoke their pipes and chew tobacco. Often the stories were in appropriate for children to hear. This made it all the more interesting for the children. In the summertime the awning would be lowered to keep the sun out of the display window and shelter these same men, who would gather on the front porch to tell the same stories and watch the local color go by. They were especially interested in the young girls and women who might venture into the store to make purchases.

As these colorful local characters would assemble on the bench in the summer and around the stove in the winter, each man had his particular point to make. The discussions could get loud, long, and at times profane. Among others, topics discussed by those sitting on the bench or around the stove included local politics, the weather, and speculations about whether the crops were going to produce as well as they did last year.

The loafers were primarily nonbelievers or members of the local Roman Catholic Church. It was a small congregation, and the priest served it along with another group nearby.

In the summer it was my responsibility to walk the half mile to the store to purchase our needs, dodging the dogs as I walked. Each farm or home along the gravel road had a dog to protect the property. In the wintertime, Dad would drive his Model A Ford to this store to make our purchases.

The country store—long may it live.

White Swan Hotel

AFTER A RAINY ride up the Pearl River, we arrived in Guangzhou, China, a city about seventy-five miles northwest of Hong Kong. Taxis carried our thirty-five persons, plus five children, to the White Swan Hotel, where we were to meet our sponsoring school representatives.

Tall buildings are commonplace in the Hong Kong area, and the hotel was no exception. This white structure stood out in contrast to the many small, low-hung buildings surrounding it.

We looked like a ragged group of peasants coming into the hotel. The White Swan was and is a gathering place for the rich and famous who make their homes in Guangzhou when they are there on business. It was possible for us to be there because of the director of the English, teaching operation over many areas of China. He was in and out of the White Swan as he worked with the different schools and colleges in the People's Republic. Large corporations, especially oil companies, kept suites of rooms for their top employees. These were rented on an annual basis. Thus, the director had access to certain suites when he was in the city because of his connection with certain executives of the oil corporation, which had its home base in Tulsa. We needed a place to connect with the educational, institutional representatives we were to meet. So the director of the institute took advantage of his Tulsa friendship, utilizing their facilities as needed.

We had eaten only a very light breakfast before being hurried out of our hotel rooms in Hong Kong that morning, so we were all hungry, especially the children. After we arrived, we were ushered into the dining room of the hotel. We were amazed to see a well-decorated room. Of course, we did not have anything to compare it with since the hotels in which we'd stayed in Hong Kong were modest rooms. We had no idea of the affluence of the folks in that area. Later on, during a return trip, I saw the magnificence of a hotel near where we had stayed in Hong Kong with Rolls-Royces and Mercedes automobiles parked out front and paid drivers seated in the cars, because this was the only place where they could be parked.

It was February of 1967, and the weather in Guangzhou was very different from the weather we had left in Tulsa, Oklahoma. In Tulsa it had been cold and miserably damp with some snow on the ground. In this city it was also cold and damp, but as we sat in the dining room of the hotel, the sun began to shine through the large windows.

Not knowing what to expect as far as the weather, we did not have the proper clothing for the winter climate in Guangzhou, which is situated on the Pearl River just off the Pacific Ocean. Strong winds and rain are common in this city, just as in Hong Kong and Macao (another city close by).

For those of us who were going to all types of institutions in China with different accommodations, being at the White Swan was a pleasurable experience. Many of us wished we could stay there overnight, but this was not to be. Our representatives from the different educational institutions began arriving; soon we were on our way to many different regions in Mainland China.

If you are ever in Guangzhou, visit the White Swan Hotel.

Grandma Was a Preacher

IT WAS SUNDAY morning in a village church in a small town in central Michigan. I was sitting in the pew with my grandfather at the end, where I could see the central figure as I looked toward the pulpit. It was my grandmother. (This small denomination ordained both men and women as preachers.)

Grandmother and her first husband, who had died in an accident several years previously, had been a working team. Later in her life she married my step-grandfather, the only person I ever knew as Grandfather.

Many years earlier, my paternal grandmother and grandfather had ministered on the prairies of Alberta, Canada. They were missionaries for their church to the settlers on the open land; the land became yours after you lived on it for a certain number of years.

When grandfather moved to Canada, he brought with him a team of horses and certain equipment to set up a farming operation. It was common in the early years of the twentieth century for ministers in this small denomination to be farmers or to have other occupations by which they earned their living. Over a period of years, my grandparents built a farmhouse, a barn, and the usual outbuildings used in that open country. Also, they had been able to purchase a cow, which they had bred, and she produced calves.

In the summertime Grandfather would farm six hundred acres of wheat land; in the wintertime he would pastor persons of his denomination. The services were held in the schoolhouses scattered over the prairies.

Grandmother was a housewife, rearing their young son who had been born to my grandparents while they still lived in Michigan. Now she was the central figure in keeping the farm and her child headed in the proper direction. While Grandfather was out and about, Grandmother kept the farming operation going, using a hired hand to do the heavy work, which she or her young son could not accomplish.

As a child sitting in the end pew of this village church, I knew none of this history. It wasn't until years later that I learned the history, which I have related, from my grandmother and my father.

My grandmother had a tremendous amount of influence in my young life and in the early years of my maturing. She was the essence of love as far as I was concerned. Her love for me was unconditional. Perhaps it was because my first breath was taken in the front bedroom of her home in Hastings, Michigan. Of course, my mother was doing the birthing with the aid of the family doctor, and she played an even greater role in my later years of life, defending me when my father wanted to "kick" me out of the house.

These two women taught me the meaning of unconditional love. It is not to say that they never guided my actions, for this they did. I was not allowed to run over them. Mother and Grandmother saw to it that my discipline was carried out but with love.

In the Depression years, my grandmother was assigned to a congregation in a small city. She never drove a car; thus, her visitation to the families of her group was accomplished by walking. She attempted to see that members of her congregation had help in meeting their bills and in having food to eat. This was no small task for this lady who was now in her late sixties. She was devoted to her calling until she died after being retired for twenty years and living on her small savings and a pension that the state of Michigan had set in motion.

Did my grandmother have personality difficulties? Yes. Even though she was my beloved grandmother, she was also a human being with faults common to humankind. But Grandmother was a preacher, a "servant of God." He was always the center of her life. She had a personal relationship with Jesus Christ.

In my late life, the picture of my grandmother in the pulpit is still fresh in my memory. She was a very able preacher and conducted the worship services in a professional manner. Her prayers are still fresh in my mind, as she would begin, "Our heavenly Parent..." She was way ahead of the current crop of pastors, who are only now coming to understand God as both male and female. The males could not bring themselves to see God as a complete person. Their eyes were blinded as to His personality. Their maleness closed their spiritual eyes to that which He really was. Yes, Grandmother was a preacher.

My First Car

DO YOU REMEMBER your first car? I imagine you do. Was it a "cheapy" or very expensive, that is, according to your income at the time? Did you believe it would be your last car or that it was just a beginner? Everyone remembers his or her first automobile.

The fall of 1938 I had to begin driving ten miles each way to get to high school. My grandmother purchased a 1929 Model T Ford for this purpose at a cost of $25. At that time, my family did not have this amount of money to buy even a cheap vehicle for me to drive. With five children to feed on the salary of a country minister, nothing extra was available.

To help meet the purchase price of gasoline, three female students rode with me five days a week to the school in the city of Fowlerville, Michigan. They paid a small amount to ride, but it was enough to buy the needed fuel.

To this day, I can still remember my first driving lesson with my father down US 16, starting out in the city of Fowlerville. Father sat beside me and instructed me in pushing the proper pedals to cause the transmission to engage as needed.

You need to know that I had never previously driven an automobile. Finally, I was able to get my feet coordinated, and we started down the highway. As we traveled down the city streets, I noticed a dog and looked to see what it was doing. Of course, the car began to follow the dog. My father noted what was happening and called out, "Lyle, look where you're driving." When I looked up, we were headed across the other lane, and fortunately no other car was in that lane. Since that day seventy years ago, my attention has always been fixed on where I am going when I'm in the driver's seat.

Today it would be necessary for me to take driver's training before I even would be granted a learner's permit. How wise we are in this day. Still, even with driver's training, many students are involved in automobile wrecks.

Today it also would be necessary for me to have auto insurance before attempting to drive. However, many persons driving in this city do not have auto insurance. This is one of the reasons our rates are so high. We, who do carry auto insurance, pay for those individuals who have no insurance.

Back to my first car—the '29 Model T Ford had two doors and two front seats that folded up to allow passengers to enter the rear full seat. This gave me room to drive the three females to school. One of the female passengers was always late when we stopped at her home. She never seemed to be able to get herself together. To help in this effort, I made it my plan to pick her up as the last person in our group. It never failed; she still wasn't ready. I wonder if she was late to her own wedding.

The country roads we navigated were often very rutted and difficult to drive on. The wise action was to get in the rut and stay there until it was time to turn out to arrive at your destination. The Model T had a rather unforgiving steering mechanism, so it was easy to lose control of the machine in such situations.

One day while driving down the country road to pick up two of the girls, sisters, chickens were in the ruts. Not wanting to attempt to turn out of the ruts, I ran over three chickens. The females were very upset with me. Whether they ever recovered from that incident is questionable.

At the young age of fourteen, what they thought did not make much sense to me. Today, I would be very unhappy to commit such an act. At that time, these chickens were very valuable, and it would have been easy for me to have honked my horn at the birds until they got out of the way.

The age of fourteen is not too wise.

For example, one winter day the young men were doing driving exercises on the slippery ice. Not wanting to be outdone, I was driving the Model T as fast as it would go on the ice, then turning the wheels abruptly to the left, which spun the car around on the ice. This happened only a few times before the superintendent of the high school came out and told me in no uncertain terms to "stop, NOW!"

Such actions rate as stupid! Many of my driving experiences were not too intelligent. Perhaps I thought as my grandson did. He told me one day, "Grandpa, we are invincible."

At the end of the first year of my driving back and forth twenty miles a day, the '29 Model T was finished. Working that summer, and making a trade-in of the Model T, I purchased a Model A coupe with a rumble seat.

My first car was finished.

Living on the Corner

HAVE YOU EVER lived on the corner of a street? For five years the family that I grew up in lived on the corner of a dusty highway. In 1933 our family moved to a parsonage on the corner of a busy country road. Vehicles traveled this highway going to and from the main business districts of central Michigan. Both districts are cities now, but more than likely, they would have been considered large villages in 1933.

Our family of seven lived on this corner. Like I said, traffic was busy for a country highway. One-half mile north of us was a small village named Cohocatah Center; three miles from our home was a larger village called Cohocatah. By these names you will note that we lived in what had been Native American land. The early settlers in Michigan had pushed the natives out and on to reservations.

As to living on the corner, once the east/west road had intersected a north/south road, as if you were crossing an intersection. In our time the east/west road had been made into a curve on the corner of the two highways. They were both gravel roads, and dust was a regular item with which to contend. My mother was always in the process of cleaning our house of the dust.

In the wintertime, dust was not the problem; it then became mud. Michigan is noted for its rain and snow and its many dark, sunless days. My uncle once said, "Michigan's weather was eight months of rain and snow with four months of summer that included abundant rain." To add to the dreary weather or to the appearance of it, around the parsonage were tall maple trees. These provided shelter from the hot sun in the summer, but in the winter they added to the gloom of the corner.

Living on this corner, we saw all kinds of life take place. We saw trucks hauling animals to market, families driving to the stores in either of the two small villages or the larger cities south of our home, and many different folks walking on this dusty road. Not everyone had a vehicle to travel to the small villages nearby.

Of course, there were also the times when the undertakers in the cities traveled past our home with their hearses. This took on a somber note when the vehicle drew up to the small church on the corner, where my father was the pastor and the parsonage was located. This took on a special note of grieving when my high school friend was killed in an automobile accident on his way home. The memorial service was held in the small church on the corner. All the members of the church attended the memorial service. Life for me was not the same for a number of weeks, especially when, on my way to high school, I drove past the corner, where he was killed.

For three years prior to my driving to high school, my two brothers and sisters and I attended the one-room country school located a quarter of a mile south of the parsonage. Here we learned the basics of education common to the country schools of the 1930s. It was from this school that I graduated from the eighth grade. And after passing the county educational exams, I was allowed to register for high school. You see, educational exams for entrance to a higher educational facility were present seventy years ago.

From this corner our family lived and visited with other children in the area. To find many children, you needed to travel to one of the two small villages mentioned in the first portion of this article. We did have one male friend who lived about halfway to the country school. He was an only child. We two older boys would play with him.

Even without lots of other children around, our family had plenty of excitement all by ourselves. Five children, ranging in age from three months to eleven years, kept the corner occupied with the usual family fights that happen between kids. I was thirty-eight months older than my next sibling, my sister. She was thirteen months older than our brother and five years older than our sister. Our youngest brother was eleven years younger than I. There was always excitement on the corner.

Do you have memories of living on a corner?

On the Cutting Edge

MY GRANDFATHER ALWAYS wanted to be on the cutting edge. When free land was being given away in Canada in 1905, he decided this was for him. Consequently, he homesteaded six hundred acres of prairie land near Lethbridge, Ontario. As an ordained minister he would farm in the summer and preach after his crops were harvested. In the wintertime he would travel from schoolhouse to schoolhouse, holding religious services.

Before going to Canada, Grandfather had lived with relatives for several years in western Kansas. He went there to cure his TB, which he contracted from his first wife, who died after one year of marriage. She had the disease and did not know it when they married.

Grandfather had an adventurous nature, always looking for the next exciting move. His church wanted an ordained minister to move to Canada and plant churches, so he accepted the challenge. Selling all his possessions in Michigan, he engaged a boxcar, loaded his team of horses, a buggy, some few items of furniture he could carry, and food for the team. He slept in one end of the boxcar, enabling him to care for his horses as they traveled by rail to Lethbridge, Canada.

Arriving in Lethbridge, he built a "soddy" for himself and began to contact persons who were members of the denomination with which he was affiliated. This involved traveling many miles with his horse and buggy and living with the persons who were of his denomination.

Soon he began to have different groups gathering in the schoolhouses for worship on Sundays. Over the years, many groups were formed. When he left eleven years later, several congregations were growing in each prairie community.

Meanwhile, his wife and young son were waiting in Michigan for him to send word for them to come and be with him. No word came. My grandmother, also a forward soul, took matters in hand, purchased rail tickets to Lethbridge, and arrived there one evening. She had sent word by letter as to the day she and her young son would arrive. Upon their arrival, no grandfather was present to greet them. They waited and waited, but still no grandfather appeared.

Because Lethbridge was a very small place at that time, grandmother inquired about where her husband's "soddy" was located and proceeded to go there. Upon her arrival, she found the house padlocked. A neighbor arrived with a pitchfork and proceeded to pull the lock off the door. Grandmother and son made themselves at home, such as they could in a bachelor's quarters.

Somehow word came to Grandfather that his wife and young son were in his home in Lethbridge. Grandfather arrived a day or two later, explaining that she and their son had arrived before her letter. When this marital matter was settled, Grandfather did his best to make his wife and son at home in his "soddy." Grandmother and son lived in this arrangement for several years until he could accumulate enough money to build a decent house on the land he homesteaded.

Soon, back on the trail Grandfather went to the land where he was tilling and planting a wheat crop because it was springtime. Meanwhile, Grandmother and my father lived in the village. She acquired a cow and began selling milk, cheese, and butter.

Chinese persons lived in Lethbridge and ran laundries, restaurants, and other services. It was my father's responsibility to carry the dairy products to the different outlets, many of them run by the Chinese males. They made much of him, but the strange-looking men frightened my father because he was only a little boy. No longer did he desire to carry the dairy products to different customers. This was his first encounter with the public.

In a few years the family moved to the six hundred acres Grandfather had claimed, and their village activities ceased. Now Grandmother took care of their child and home, while Grandfather continued his traveling ministry in the wintertime and farming in the summer.

Their son began his education in the Canadian school system, which was based on the educational system from the United Kingdom. He had a good foundation for later experiences after his parents returned to live in Michigan.

In the early years of our nation, it was common for ministers to farm and, in addition, carry on their ministries. Most congregations had very little cash income; thus, the minister was forced to earn the majority of his income from secular work. In some areas of the world today, this is still the pattern of life.

Many pastors still live on the edge, not the cutting edge, but many of them live on the edge of poverty.

On Taking a Bath

"CLEANLINESS IS NEXT to godliness." We children thought this was our mother's motto. She was a crank about her children being immaculate. Mom made sure each of us was as clean as possible on the salary of a very poorly paid preacher. Perhaps she was making up for the poverty income our father was paid by the churches he served.

A large cake of Ivory soap was the standard used to keep us children smelling properly. Now this was no small job with five children to keep on the cleanliness train. Our usual Saturday night ritual was to bathe in the circular washtub. If you have never washed in the galvanized, circular tub, you have missed a treat. The rest of the week Mom washed our assorted clothes in the tub. (It seemed she was always doing the washing. We were always heating water on the kitchen stove.) But Saturday night, the tub was ours.

"Wash your neck" was a command Mom made to us boys, all three of us. What she told the girls, well, I do not know that command.

This concept of staying clean has carried over into my adult life. I need to be clean, not excessively so, but clean. Smelly people are anathema to me.

Salt and Pepper

For several summers my wife and I performed volunteer work in the parks of the state of Oregon and were hosts in the lighthouses on the coast. Being in a confined area, as different groups came up the stairs of the structures, I came to know the types of people who were coming. Many of the foreign folk use no deodorant; they seem to enjoy the body odors. It took only one whiff to know we were entertaining people from another culture. However, I must say, campers are not always clean-smelling people either, no matter where they come from. Now I am in real trouble with campers, right?

Back to my family cleanliness project or, I should say, Mom's campaign to keep her children clean. She had an impossible job, dealing with limited bathing facilities.

Think of heating the bathwater on top of a coal-burning kitchen stove. Also, we had to pump the water outside the house, carry it inside, and fill the tub. Then we carried the dirty water outside, dumped it, and refilled the galvanized tub for the next body to be scrubbed. Quite literally, it was scrubbed. With a washrag and Ivory soap—the large bar—Mom scrubbed us, that is, until we were old enough to do the job ourselves. That is when the command came from Mom. "Wash your neck!"

The youth of our day, with our modern facilities, have no idea how difficult it was to keep the "smellies" under control. With the advent of modern plumbing, everything changed. The majority of people now have the availability of facilities to keep themselves clean.

Still, I wonder how many mothers still have to check on their sons to see if they have washed their necks.

Women Who Have Influenced My Life

CAN YOU NAME the women who have influenced your life? Three have been major factors in my life. They are my mother, grandmother, and wife. These three women have loved me in their own individual ways.

As I was the first child born to my mother, it appears she always had a special place in her heart for me. Mother defended me against my father, when in one of his angry moments he was throwing me out of the house. My mother told him, "Paul, if he leaves, I leave also." He didn't throw me out because he would have had to take care of four other children all by himself. Even to this day—and she has been dead since 1998—I can feel the touch of my mother's hands and the way she held me in her arms.

Grandmother came into my life the day I was born. This took place eighty-six years ago when the medical doctor in the front bedroom of her home delivered me. She seemed to have a special affection for this man-child until the day she died at the age of eighty-seven. Each month, at least, we would exchange a letter. When I was in college, from her meager income she would send me money to help me pay my expenses.

Salt and Pepper

Both Grandmother and Mother took care of me when I had scarlet fever and a relapse at the age of eighteen months. They were confined in the same house under the state-demanded quarantine until the medical doctor released me.

My wife and I washed dishes together in the kitchen of the small college we attended in Indiana. This was before the state health department demanded mechanical, sterilized dish washing.

In college we earned our way. First we were given the jobs of washing dishes, pots and pans, and whatever else the head cook needed. Later on, my wife worked in the college library, and I had the position as one of the janitors, cleaning rooms and bathrooms.

Both of us knew dish washing from the duties we had experienced in our homes. We were the eldest children in our families—she in a family of three, and I in a family of five. As early as five years old, she had stood on a wooden box and washed dishes. I had begun this chore when my mother was overwhelmed with four other children.

Of course, as we washed and dried the dishes, we talked. Slowly, the lady who was to become my wife one and a half years later worked her way into my emotions. After we were married years later, she told me, "When I saw you the first time, I was determined to marry you."

My wife has been my best friend and lover for sixty-six years. She loved me when giving birth to our three children. She loved me when I was ill after several operations, including one that was very serious, in which she took care of me for five weeks as I recovered from severe surgery. She showed her love when I was close to dying while on a trip to China, where she found me flopped in the bathtub in the hotel where we were staying. She gave to me by sharing her body as we made love and produced three children. Never once has she said, "No!" This lovely creature has showered blessings upon me.

As I have wandered from place to place over our married life, only once has she raised objection to the place where we were living. As we were driving out of this hole in the ground in southwestern Colorado, she told me, "If it is all right with you, don't bring me back to a place like this to live."

Now in our mid-eighties, we take care of each other. Both my mother and grandmother have long been in their eternal home. My wife continues to be my lover, best friend, and the one I can trust with my deepest thoughts.

I am a blessed man with three women who have influenced my life. Each of them loved and loves me in her own individual way.

Scared Stiff

IN THE SUMMER of 1929 I was staying at my grandmother's home in Baltimore, Michigan. Being a child of seven years, my imagination ran wild at the slightest strange sound.

There were only the three of us in the whole house. It was a large house with many windows. The rooms were large, and at night it seemed every room was occupied by strange sounds. Around the large, two-story brick farmhouse were tall evergreen trees. These trees were very old, perhaps native to the area. At night the wind would whistle through the trees with a moaning sound. When the wind would moan like this through the trees, I would become paralyzed with fear; it scared me stiff.

Normally I was required to sleep upstairs, and my grandparents slept downstairs. But because I was so frightened, my grandparents allowed me to sleep on a couch in the living room. Here I could be close to them and be assured of their presence by their snoring.

As I lay on the couch in the living room, strange sights would appear in the windows as the moon thrust its shadows through the glass. Of course, a little boy's imagination was in full play. All types of persons were lurking outside the window, such as robbers, murderers, and even those who would kidnap a small, defenseless boy.

Each night I stayed awake as long as possible with the lamps burning so that it would be impossible for harm to take me. As long as the lamp was burning, it seemed to me that no harm could overtake me. Of course, it was impossible for the kerosene lamp to be kept burning all night. The possibility of fire was ever present.

My grandfather, really my step-grandfather, had reared two children in this house. His first wife had died, and he married my grandmother after her husband, my grandfather, was killed in an accident.

At one time this brick farmhouse had been envied by other farmers in the area. The family had been early settlers in Baltimore Township. The father had provided each of the sons a large acreage and the same to his only daughter and her husband. The family had been substantial in the community at one time. Those days were gone with the crash of 1929. Farmers in the area were just hanging on financially.

Of course, this child never sensed the money problems. All he worried about was the strange noises that came around the house at night when he was placed in bed and told to go to sleep and that nothing would harm him. Even after his "Now I lay me down to sleep" prayer, the strange noises still existed. His grandmother told him God was there and nothing could harm him, but to this small child, God was far away. God seemed to be unaware of the fear in the mind of a seven-year-old with a large imagination.

Thus, Grandmother made it possible for her grandson, the apple of her eye, to sleep on the couch in the living room. Noises were still present, and strange lights flashed through the large front windows, but the snoring of grandparents in the next room made the little boy feel much more secure than in an upstairs bedroom far away from protection.

Can you remember when you were a small child and had an experience such as this, or one similar? I believe all children have similar experiences. This is why parents keep an electric light burning in the room of a child who has a strong imagination. This eases the fears of the child, and then the mother and father can get a good night of rest.

Sunday

AS A CHILD I hated to see Sunday come. We were preacher's kids; our activities were confined to reading the Bible, our story leaflet from Sunday school, or some other religious book—no games at all. Mom would not hear of such action on the Lord's Day. We children could and did chase each other around in the yards surrounding the parsonage and church building, but that was it. Oh, yes, and we did fight with each other because of having nothing else to do. Mom would allow us to sleep if we needed it. Dad would have been more open to our doing something, just anything, but Mom would not allow it.

Sunday…we children often wondered what other kids did on that day. Of course, the farm kids had chores to do and did them, no questions asked: milking cows, feeding chickens, and slopping the pigs. The farm children only had one change from their regular routine; they would attend morning worship and Sunday school and go to an evening worship service or Christian Endeavor, if they were older.

We longed for Monday morning to arrive. Off to school, a one-room country school. We walked, no buses, and on a cold January morning in Michigan, you walked as rapidly as you could to get to school. At least Sunday was over for another week.

Sunday morning in the winter was another battle. Because our family lived next door to the church building, it was our duty to start the fire in the furnace long before the service began to warm the old building up, as it had been closed all week except for a prayer meeting on Wednesday evening. When we children were small, Dad had to build the fire before he drove to another church for a worship service. When we were old enough to be trusted, it became our duty—I should say *my* duty—to build the fire. I was the eldest child in our family.

I had to be very careful not to build too much of a fire at first because the furnace would smoke, and the congregation did not like to breathe smoke when they came to the worship service, especially the women. It was also my duty to shovel snow off the front steps because these were not covered. This demanded getting out early and salting the steps so that the ice under the snow would melt.

From reading this little dissertation, you may gather that I despised Sundays. Oh, and not only did all of this take place, but also we children had to listen to the sermon our father preached. In this particular conservative congregation, "hell fire and brimstone" was not unusual. If you did not feel condemned after the service was finished, you felt something must be wrong with your relationship with God. For Father had his directions from God; what he preached was as if it came directly from the Father above. Who was to argue with his message? One did not argue with the representative of God on earth.

I am in no way putting God down; this was only how this particular denomination interpreted the Bible, and to some extent does to this very day. Perhaps this is why this denomination has about the same membership it had when I was a child.

Looking back on this experience has colored my understanding of Sundays. I feel very uncomfortable if I do anything that does not come under the same rules that were laid down by Mother and Father. To Mom, rest her soul in peace, Sunday was literally a day of rest, except Dad had to work very hard with two services to lead. He was really tired out when the day was over.

On the other hand, Sunday to my wife's family was very different, even within the same denomination. The Sunday school and worship rituals were the same, but the rules after the service were much different. In the afternoon, often the family would drive to the country to visit a relative, have fun with games, and eat handmade ice cream. My wife's father loved to have a good time, and he enjoyed seeing others do the same. Hard work was his lot six days per week, but on Sunday, it was time to enjoy both God and his fellowmen.

Sunday—do you have a positive memory, or is it negative?

Change

WHAT DO YOU think "change" means? The hymn goes, "Change and decay in all around I see; O Thou who changest not, abide with me."

We human beings do not look for change. We enjoy stability. We want things to remain just as they are. "Don't rock my boat," we say. Because we do not know what takes place beyond what we see, change does not appeal to human beings. Why are we this way? Because many are convinced that life does not exist beyond what the human eye can see. Life is expendable; one does not know from this day to the next whether he or she will be alive. We humans do not bother with the thought of change.

As a child it was impossible for me to envision anything beyond the present situation. Somewhere between the ages of ten and twelve years, it became possible for me to visualize change. By the time the years of accountability had arrived, my maternal grandmother had died, my aunt had died of cancer, and my delightful grandfather was left alone.

Even though I did not grieve the death of my grandmother, it became very real to me because of how it affected my mother. This sickly old lady had been the mainstay of the family. Never had I known her, except when she was ill. It was no wonder with her having birthed eight children and with seven living. As far as I could tell, all seven delighted in Grandmother.

Change occurred when Grandma died. Our regular trips to Leslie, Michigan, ceased. Before, Mother had been able to twist Dad's arm to drive her to Leslie to see Grandma. Change in this situation meant we children would not have the chance to see our cousins as often.

Change took place again. His daughters living nearby saw to it that Grandfather's only sister arrived to keep him company. The aunt became the dominant female in the household. Grandfather had someone to keep track of him, wash his clothes, and cook his meals. In addition, she was a strong Bible student, having been a member of the Volunteers of America, an organization set up like the Salvation Army. Now Grandfather had someone who would share Bible concepts with him.

Change for Grandfather meant he could now have an assistant without the tongues of the community wagging. He had been interested in a fine female from his local church, but his daughters had stopped that. So he endured aunty. Because of her presence, Granddad had a female to keep him company—a person who would attend worship services with him, pray with him, and study the Bible with him regularly.

As you may notice, change can mean many different things, depending upon the situation.

For my mother, change was rather dramatic. She went from a young single woman doing housework for others to being a wife and mother in five years. Mom suddenly had to face the demands of a husband, of a mother-in-law, and finally, of having five children in a period of eleven years. Also, she had to live on the up-and-down income Dad received from the congregations he served. Dad was supposed to receive a salary, but it depended upon how generous the members of the churches were or how their crops prospered or the level of their milk checks.

Change on Father's side of the family was depressing because he had always been able to fall back on the money Grandmother gave him each time he visited her. But in the Depression, the financial outlook was bleak. The small amount of income she received from her rented house depended upon whether or not the renter worked. My step-grandfather's income depended upon the ability of the farm renter to pay as promised. Both grandparents had property but little income.

Change at this time, in the depths of the Depression, meant a growing number of the elderly were on very limited incomes. To help this situation, the legislature passed an act to pay each resident over a certain age a fixed income. In this manner, the elderly persons could have enough to pay for some food and fuel and to give a little to their particular charity.

Change; let us hope this does not take place again.

Section Two

Family Life

Downhill Slide

AS A SIX-YEAR-OLD boy, sliding downhill on a large sled was thrilling. The place was New Dundee, Ontario, Canada. It was winter, and the snow was slick on the long hill that ran through the center of town. Even the older boys, almost men, delighted in sliding down the hill as fast as they could propel their sleds.

One time, I was invited by an older male to slide down the hill with him. The operation went like this: he would begin his run to gather up speed, and I was to jump on his back at the very last minute.

Success! I made the jump, landed on his back, and zoomed down the hill at lightning speed. When I opened my eyes, dismay chilled me. We were traveling at a tremendous speed down a hill with other boys on sleds flashing by us and the bottom of the hill rushing toward us. Never had I traveled at such speed toward the end of who knows where. And to top this journey off, I knew we had to successfully pass through the walls of a bridge that covered the stream running through the town.

Can you picture this feeling? No way could I control what was happening. I was completely at the mercy of the older male who was steering the sled. The air was rushing past my face at breakneck speed. What was I to do? Screaming would not help. The sled was traveling too quickly for me to jump off. So I closed my eyes, hoping the older boy would know what to do to steer through the walls of the bridge.

All at once we sprang through the sides of the bridge and came to a level spot, which slowed the sled down almost immediately. After we stopped and I was able to stand up, the thrill of the experience caused me to want to do it all over again. Now it was necessary to walk back up the long hill to begin the journey again.

In the years ahead, sledding was a common bit of fun, but never again did I have the thrill that went with this lightning speed ride I experienced on the back of another male on a sled, at night, on a snow-packed road.

When was the last time you had a thrill such as the one described above? Did you ever have this experience, or did you have one much more thrilling than this? Sled rides are thrilling. Each one has its own particular story to tell. Can you match this incident?

Perhaps this story will cause you to remember an incident such as this that occurred in your life. Why not write it down and give it to your children, or perhaps sell it to some newspaper or magazine? Better yet, keep it in your memory to tell to a boy who is looking for a thrill.

Here in Arizona, it would be necessary to travel up the mountains or to the northern part of the state, where seven to eight feet of snow fall each winter, to even try sledding. But it can still be done, even in desert country. Looking for a challenge? There you have it.

Mourning Doves

JUST NOW, LOOKING out our front door and watching two mourning doves, they remind me of the verses in Matthew 19:4–6, where Jesus is reported to have said, “Haven’t you read that at the beginning the Creator ‘made them male and female,’ and said, ‘For this reason a man will leave his father and mother and be united to his wife, and the two will become one flesh’? So they are no longer two, but one. Therefore what God has joined together, let man not separate.”

In my reading, it appears that the mourning doves become one. They stay together all through their fowl life. As I watched these birds, if one of them got over the fence, the other one became very frustrated and attempted to be with his or her mate.

If God made birds to be life partners, why do humans leave their partners for other partners?

In my years of counseling, listening to the heartbreak of people as they exchanged partners, I saw how true the Scripture is. In listening to the woes of husbands and wives, they tell me again and again, after they recover from their anger, “I was a fool not to have stayed with my first love.”

Salt and Pepper

A well-known politician, writing his thoughts, stated, "It was my fault the first marriage did not work." Lesser folks sharing their souls in counseling have stated this same truism.

In our present-day society, we change partners as easily as we change our clothes. The state laws assist us in this process. But God did not ordain one man and one woman for each other for life to take the fun out of changing partners. He knew we are made to find our satisfaction with our first love. We may be sexually attracted to another person, and that attraction may send us into a passion tizzy, but such a lust is not true love.

Real love is founded upon what we can do for the other individual in the marriage. The mourning doves seek to share everything they find together. If one finds a source of food, he or she calls the mate to partake. They find comfort in sharing.

After sixty-six years of marriage to the same female, I am beginning to learn what true love is. At first the attraction was pure lust, but later on it became a sense of two souls united and working for the good of the couple. We left our parents and became one, not all at once, but over the years, each of us attempting to assist the other in finding love in the relationship. Today we find we are often saying to each other "thank you" and "please," even as we would to a total stranger.

In our society this sense of pleasure in your mate is often lacking. We males especially forget the attitude we expressed to our mate when we were dating her once she takes on our name. We take each other for granted.

The other evening at the evening meal, my wife and I were discussing this problem. Both of us acknowledged that we did not cherish each other as we should. The years seem to have worn off the edges of courtesy.

We are now in our mid-eighties; time is running out for us to be together as one flesh. Perhaps this is why we take note of our lack of correctness with each other, or maybe it is more than correctness; perhaps it is that we do not seem to sense that both of us are partners in our marriage.

Mourning Doves

Each day we attempt to kiss and hold each other, knowing that one day in the next few years one of us will leave and the other partner will be alone, remembering how we missed such opportunities.

In the evening I see one dove fly in and rest on the electric wire outside my window. Soon the mate swoops in and cuddles up to its mate.

We could learn a lesson from the mourning dove couple, right?

Babies

DID YOU EVER wonder what you looked like on the day you were born? Many of us have only what our mother tells us about how we looked. Of course, according to her you were the most adorable being ever given to womankind.

In my case, apparently the neighbor living next door to my grandmother's house was so interested in seeing my birth that she was found in the bushes underneath the window of the bedroom where the event was taking place.

All this brings me to comment on the beauty of babies. There is a certain delicious smell about a little one, that is, until the little one learns to "poop" in his or her pants. That smell is not delicious. Only a mother and a few fathers can appreciate that odor. Notwithstanding, there is a certain beauty about newborn children—their curly hair or their ten fingers, the wiggle of their ten toes, and the belly breathing... seeing the tiny chest move in and out as if some mysterious inner control was at work.

Yesterday, I saw a four-month-old only child. His eyes seemed to take in every movement. His blue eyes sparkled as he looked at all the excitement of his new surroundings. As you see this in the face and eyes of a child, you wonder what is taking place in the tiny brain.

When the baby looked at his mother, you could see a certain recognition of her as someone he could and wanted to relate to. As he continued to look at her, a tiny smile began to occur in the corners of his mouth. She was the person he could trust, for he had learned over the past four months that she was the security blanket he needed at all times. Trust blossomed in his face. She could be counted on to see his needs fulfilled, even as she had for the nine months he was in her womb. It was the same heartbeat he knew and understood.

Only since I have exceeded my three score years and ten has the wonder of babies taken my fancy. They say babies and old men have something in common: blind, toothless, bald headed, and potbellied. Maybe this is why I now enjoy them. Or is it because I can observe and appreciate them as their parents take care of them?

I'm convinced that God knew what He was doing when He gave young adults the power to bring babies into this world. Looking back on that time in my life, I am happy for the children in our family, that their mother, my wife, was a mature twenty-two years old when she began rearing a very active son. As the father, I was always busy earning a living and attending college or graduate school.

My wife had worked for a few years with children in a family; thus, she was more adept with newborn and young children. My experience had been in assisting Mother when taking care of two brothers and two sisters. Our father was always busy with his pastoral work or growing a garden to feed five little mouths, almost as tiny birds with their beaks opened wide to catch a morsel of food.

Babies must have been a blessing God intended for parents. He stated, "Be fruitful and multiply." Some parents have taken Him at His word, and we see large families. Others in our day and time have decided to control their supply of babies and have two or three at most.

The other day twins came into the waiting room of the hospital where I do volunteer work one afternoon each week. They were four or five months old. These two little beings sparkled like fairies. Their grandmother beamed, and their mother had a smile all over her face when I paid attention to the little girl. There was a boy and a girl. They even looked alike, except for their gender difference.

Twins! What went through the mind of that mother when she was informed from an ultrasound that she was carrying twins? Perhaps: *Wow! Double blessings! Hardly. Double costs all the way from birth to the day they go out the door as young adults.*

Have you ever been in the nursery of a hospital where all the newborns are housed? What happens when one cries? A chorus begins as one newborn after another joins in the choir. Think what it would be like to have two babies crying at the same time. What could the mother do to quiet one and then the other? Perhaps thrust a bottle into the mouth of one and then the other?

Yes, babies are blessings that are especially sent from God; the only problem is that we often hurry His plans.

Imagination

MANY OF THE books by C. S. Lewis grew out of his imagination. He was a distinguished don at Cambridge University; coming from a religious background, he was then an atheist, but he then became an evangelical Christian. His books have intrigued both children and adults. It could be said that Lewis had a holy imagination. In many ways as a writer, he was a child.

Imagination allows us to regress to our childhood. Imagination allows me to travel back to my years as a child and young adult. Here I can live without adults thinking my mind has deserted me. If I talk to myself, it is not because of insanity but because imagination has taken hold of my mind for a few brief moments.

My first imaginings are of a child sitting in the pew beside Grandfather Ickes as Grandmother, the preacher, led the worship service. I can still hear her praying, saying, "Our heavenly Parent" and then going on with the morning prayer. That simple church comes into view with the hard oak seats and Grandfather allowing me to sit at the end of the pew (this enabled me to see Grandmother and what was taking place in the service).

In my imagination I see a large, brick farmhouse with many rooms. It was the home of Grandfather and Grandmother Ickes before the 1929 Depression hit and Grandfather became too old to farm. I remember the windy nights in that house, when I was allowed to sleep on a couch in the parlor, close enough to hear my grandparents snore but not in the same room with them. Here I would hear the wind howling through the tall pine trees in the front yard. As a small child, these noises frightened me. In my childhood imagination all kinds of wild beings were after me. The noises the wind made howling through the pines heightened my fears…pure imagination. But being close to my grandparents helped to calm my fears.

Imagination can be a wonderful gift, or it can be used to destroy and tear down the human soul. I wonder if some of the stories in the Old Testament are not just imagination running wild—such as the donkey talking to its owner and telling him an angel is standing in front of them and barring the roadway.

Books and movies are products of the human imagination. Perhaps some incident strikes the spark which ignites the imagination, but where does all this information we process hide?

Does imagination come from the depths of our souls? Do our souls feed into our imaginations? Often ideas spring into my conscious mind over which I seem to have no control. I wonder, *How did that get there?*

For example, last evening, as I sat eating a snack, from nowhere I could smell the cooking of real bacon in the kitchen of my grandmother. Imagination! It has been fifty years since I ate in my grandmother's dining room, but there in my imagination a whiff of bacon odor sprang full into my senses…imagination.

Now in my twilight years, reality and imagination get mixed up. Sometimes it seems as if the time is real, when in reality, it is imagination. Does this ever happen to you?

Have some fun—allow your imagination to go full speed and see what happens when you do this.

Imagination…what happens in yours?

Eating Out

OUR PHONE RANG. On the line was the voice of our eldest son. "I'm coming to town and want to take you out for dinner."

I replied, "Your mother will enjoy that."

"How about you?" he asked.

I admitted that it would be enjoyable.

An hour later our son and two of his female friends arrived. We chatted for a little while, and then he said, "OK, it's time to go. Where are we going?" We told him of our favorite place, and away we went to Furr's Cafeteria.

Today, eating out is a commonplace affair. Figures I read recently indicated that 50 percent of the funds allocated for food were spent in fast food shops and restaurants—places like Kentucky Fried Chicken, Wendy's, Golden Corral, Furr's Cafeteria, and McDonald's, to name a few.

The advent of women working has hastened the eating-out syndrome. Mom is in no mood to prepare a meal after working for eight hours in an office, driving to and from work, and thinking about what she will prepare for Dad and the kids. So off they all go to the first eating establishment that they can all agree on or that Dad and Mom decide on.

Children today become acclimated to this concept as they eat out in the school cafeteria; eating out becomes part of the regular pattern of their lives. Thus, when the children become adults, this pattern is already established in their thinking.

The advent of television has also hastened the eating-out syndrome. Who desires to leave their favorite program to go to the table? Today, food is brought to the home, and Dad or Mom pays for it. Even if Mom and Dad do prepare the meal at home, often it is taken from a box, placed in the microwave, heated, and served. It has already been cooked previously.

Things were different years ago, especially in other countries. Eating out was more of a novelty. When we lived in China for a year eighteen years ago, eating out was not a privilege in which we participated. The Chinese population at that time was only beginning to come out from under the control of poverty caused by the Mao regime. But the educational leadership was able to overcome this problem by having banquets for the foreign experts, such as my spouse and me. The Chinese made up for the skimpy menu they lived on in this manner. The president of the institution would not criticize them, even though he knew what was going on.

As a child I enjoyed eating out, especially if I was in the home of my grandmother. She always knew what a little boy enjoyed and did her best to satisfy that need.

My father, being a pastor and serving rural churches, gave us the opportunity to attend meetings where food was served. These meetings were the social gatherings for the congregations. Once in a while we were invited out for a meal but not often; who could afford to feed the pastor, his wife, and his five hungry children?

My favorite eating-out time was when the Ladies Aid Society had its monthly meeting in the home of one of the parishioners. Here other boys would also come, and we ate together and visited about concerns boys have.

Eating Out

Eating out is now the pastime of US citizens and is becoming a way of life in many other countries. In fact, people all over the world enjoy eating out. When we visited Shanghai two years ago, long lines of Chinese were lined up to eat out at McDonald's. Young people quickly adopted the foods brought at by the chain food companies, even though these foods were seasoned to the taste of a particular country.

I guess it just comes down to this: people enjoy eating out, and companies are more than willing to take their money.

Remembering

TODAY I ATTENDED the memorial service for a friend. These services are not easy on anyone. As you sit through such a service, it causes you to contemplate your own mortality. These services make you stop and realize that you are not going to live forever. Perhaps in this way, such services are of value to the human race. We know individuals die, but we do not stop to think that we shall also die. Somehow our minds shut out this hard fact: I shall die.

I know that I will die, my wife will die, and so will my sons and daughter. As an old saying goes, "Two things are for sure, death and taxes."

What further good can arise from a memorial service? Memories of the good the person has done while living on this earth. Most of us humans will never be famous or remembered beyond the edge of our own families. A few people who have benefited from our being on this earth will remember us, but after that, no one will.

Memorial services bring folks together who, for a few minutes at least, remember the deceased and share about what that person meant to them. It gives the friends of the deceased the opportunity to publicly say a few good words and speak of the fine things the one who is gone did while here. It also gives the family members the privilege of saying what they enjoyed about the person. At times, the family members by their silence can make a statement about the ill feelings they may have about the deceased. Generally, though, this is not done, or it might be like the African-American wife who, upon hearing the nice words the preacher was saying about her dead husband, stood up, saying, "Let me take a look at the man in the casket. I want to see if it is the same person I was married to."

Remembering is good for the living. Things like memorial services offer the opportunity to challenge the congregation to become aware of how others will look at them when they are memorialized. This might cause those in attendance to take a deep look at the direction their lives are taking, even if no one knows what is going on other than their family members.

When some unsavory act comes to my mind to do, remembering my family keeps me on the "straight and narrow." I do not want to be remembered by my children and wife as one who ruined their name. This has nothing to do with what God may think of me and the judgment I will come under. All too often we forget the consequences of our actions until they are over, then we hang our heads in shame, saying, "How could I have been so stupid?"

Remembering is very meaningful when I think of the acts of my grandparents; both those on the paternal and maternal side left good examples for me to follow. They were solid Christian citizens with nothing to be ashamed of. Simple folks, yes, but citizens leaving a good name.

Remembering the struggle my parents went through to help me reminds me of my duty to do the very best I can to make sure my children know of the struggles my spouse and I went through to give them the items deemed necessary for living in our society. When we set these standards, they go on to our grandchildren and great-grandchildren. When this takes place, if the children fail, it is by their own choices and not because we failed them.

Remembering is also valuable and significant for nations. Unhealthy leadership not only reflects upon the leader but also upon the nation. The members of our society will be remembered in years ahead for their faulty leading. We citizens do not know all the ins and outs of political economic realities. Even though we attempt to find the truth in each situation, often we are allowed to see only what a particular leader desires us to know. This may be the truth, or it may be a falsehood. Our nation has had some undesirable leadership over the 250 years of our democracy. Other times we have had men who did their very best to lead the nation in the best direction. Remembering, we may say, "Why did he do thus and so; look what has happened to our people."

Today, with the United States holding a dominant position in the world, more than ever we are responsible for what takes place in the global scene. It is our responsibility to think very carefully about any actions we take because the remainder of the world could prosper or suffer dire consequences based on some of these decisions.

How will our nation be remembered as historians look back over the last one hundred years? Will our record be one of doing the best for the whole world, or will we be hated as a nation looking out only for ourselves? Isn't that what nations do? Should we be any different? My hope is that the people of the world will take into account the good we attempted to accomplish.

Keys to a Successful Marriage

KEYS TO A successful marriage are found in four categories: 1) Have the same educational background as your spouse. 2) Have the same financial background as your spouse. 3) Have the same religious background as your spouse. 4) Have the same family background as your spouse.

After being married to the same spouse for sixty-six years, the above factors have proven to keep our marriage on track. This is not to say that there have not been "bumps" in the journey—that would be a lie. However, we have determined that these four principles are the determining factors in our marriage, and the marriages of other couples we know, being successful.

As one who was a psychologist and family counselor for forty-five years, I believe the above determents have proven to be true in successful marriages. The old concept that opposites make for a successful marriage has not proven to be true in my experience of counseling. The more your spouse and you are alike, the better the cement is that's holding your marriage together.

Because you are molding a new relationship in marriage, it is normal for you to experience differences of opinion. But when your spouse and you have the four similar background concepts stated above, you are more likely to be able to work out any differences experienced.

A fifth principle, which I did not name above and have kept until last, is *love*. In our society today, the concept of love is really *lust*. We men think, "If I can only get her in bed, all will be right." The women believe, "If I can only get him in bed, then he will show that he loves me." No wonder 50 percent of first-time marriages end in divorce! *Love* and *lust* are not the same. *Lust* is the animal instinct running loose. *Love* is a deep sense of being connected with the right person. For many folks, distinguishing between the two in our lust-driven generation is difficult.

When the lust wears out, and it will after a period of time, people have this concept: they do not love me. The next step is for the couple to file for divorce and both go on their way to look for new partners. The sad part of this picture is that the same issues that produced the first divorce will continue into the next marriage. Seventy-five percent of second marriages end in divorce.

The moral of the story is this: stay in your present marriage unless you are being abused and obtain excellent professional counseling, working out the problems you are having. If you are about to enter into a marriage, be sure to take into account the five suggestions offered in this article.

Have a successful marriage—you are capable, and God made you that way.

Visitors

AS YOU WATCH couples around you, what are your reactions to their arrangements? Over the years, we have had many visitors to our home. Let me tell you about a few of them and share my observations.

She is twenty-nine, and he only recently turned thirty-five. What will their marriage become?

It appears, according to articles I have read, that older women are marrying younger men. Why is this phenomenon occurring? Is it because younger men are able to sexually satisfy older women better than men their own age? This is possible because older men lose their sexual abilities.

She is sixty-one, and he is fifty-nine. Why did this marriage take place? If you asked them, the answer might be that lust crept in, and they, being reared in a strict Protestant background, married before intercourse caught them. It could be that the slight age span did not matter because of the attraction in this instance. They believed in love, and the love bug captured them. They have now been married for thirty-four years. Today, if a marriage holds up more than ten years, it is doing well.

A couple visited over the Christmas season. They are both retired majors in the US Army with twenty years of service. She has a master's degree in nursing and he a master's degree in economics. Presently, they are both working in a school system; she is a school nurse, and he is teaching mathematics in a middle school in New Mexico. Currently, they are in their twenty-second year of marriage. She had a son prior to her current marriage, and he had no children from his first marriage.

Another person was present this Christmas season, a male who was sixty-three years old. He was in education for twenty-five years, the last fourteen years as an assistant principal and principal of a middle school in western Arizona. His first marriage, on the rebound, lasted ten years, and they had two children. After she walked out on him, he declared it was enough, and they divorced. Sixteen years later, he remarried. This lasted for one and a half years. Then she told him, "I love you, but I don't want to live with you." She carried out the divorce proceedings. They were both of the same age at this time.

Why do some marriages persevere and others fall by the wayside? If I could predict how a marriage would turn out, I would become a very rich man, and many persons would not have to go through the heartache attached to divorce. Children would not become the football between parents, and the family structure of our nation would be greatly improved.

Of the four couples, three had divorces, one female had a son out of wedlock, and in one marriage the children split between their parents. The boy lived with his father, who never remarried. The girl went with her mother, stating, "My mother needs me." The parents of the boy and girl lived in the same city, and the children would see each other and even went to school together. The son has been married two times and is now divorced. The girl lived with two males in college, married one of them, and they are now parents of a boy and girl. When I look at situations like this I think, *Why do we act as we do and then wonder what has taken place?*

As you can see, the background of people who visit is most interesting. When I see some of these people's struggles, I am even more grateful for how God has preserved our marriage…

Visitors

She is eighty-eight, and he is eighty-six. They were married the second year in college and became parents the next year. Today she has the equivalent of a master's degree, and he has an EdD. in educational psychology/counseling. How has their marriage survived? Perhaps because they both came from the same denominational background, economic status, and educational aspirations.

Wives Choose Husbands' Clothes

DOES YOUR WIFE choose your clothes? It is reported that many wives choose the clothes their husbands wear. Do men choose the clothes their wives wear? Have you seen a survey concerning this question? There probably is such a survey, but I have not seen it.

Many men do not really care about the clothes they wear as long as they are a good fit. Men enjoy good quality if they have the money to purchase shirts, ties, and suits. Men want an excellent fit in their shoes. We spend all day on our feet, and a good fit in shoes makes a vast difference in how a man feels at the close of the day.

The wife delights in seeing her man well dressed, just as a man delights in seeing his wife in pleasing clothes. The sales people know this and do all they can to direct the wife in choosing clothes that accent the qualities of her man. At times this is difficult because many men have physical deformities that make fitting them a problem.

As a man delights in seeing his wife well-dressed, so does the wife enjoy seeing her man in quality clothes that accent his uniqueness. Each individual has certain qualities of his or her physique that can he highlighted. All too often we forget these qualities that need to be accented. Thus, the wife, in choosing to dress her husband, needs to look for those features that will set him apart from the common run of males. A seasoned clothing clerk will size up the situation and proceed to suggest clothes that will give his or her client a distinctive appeal.

My cousin sold clothes for J.C. Penney while attending college. Using some of the principles mentioned above, he became a success in the business, earning enough to pay his way. He was a jolly type of fellow and really enjoyed people. Later in life he was both a minister and the principal of a school in Maryland. The qualities of salesmanship he learned on the floor of J.C. Penney assisted him in these occupations.

It is stated, "Clothes make the man." This is only true if the person inside is a quality individual before the clothes are draped over his body. If he is not a quality person, no amount of money spent on clothing him will make up for the poor quality of the soul inside his body.

Have you ever met a male who was well dressed but had a personality that tended to drive people away? As you looked into his eyes, what did you see? Did you see a person who could not be trusted? Was he too jolly, hiding the real person under the disguise of clothes? Could he look you in the eye, or was he always looking away?

One characteristic I look for in a well dressed man is eyes that engender trust. If his eyes betray trust, then it is my reaction to deal as little as possible with him. If he gives me a "fish handshake," at once a lack of trust registers in me, and I consider this in my dealings with him. I desire to have as little as possible, if anything, to do with this type of person. His clothes cannot cover up his lack of a trustworthy personality.

How does his wife cover up this lack of quality in this person? Perhaps this did not exist in him when the wife first married the man. Perhaps this flaw in his character has developed over a period of years. Perhaps it was always there, but he kept it hidden, and the young wife did not sense this flaw or felt she could remake his character. Sorry to say, remaking a man or woman is generally unsuccessful. When you marry a man or woman, remember. "What you see is what you get." Change, if at all possible, comes very slowly and often not at all.

Wives Choose Husbands' Clothes

Ladies, when you dress your man, look for the qualities you can accent. Thus, your man will be recognized for the person he is, not for the clothes he wears. Nice try, wives.

Thanksgiving Dinner at Grandma's House

CAN YOU REMEMBER the times you ate Thanksgiving dinner at Grandma's house? What was it like? Let me tell you about eating Thanksgiving dinner in my grandmother's house.

In the early years of my life, Thanksgiving was a time of family reunion. All the aunts, uncles, and cousins would arrive. Each family would bring enough food to feed a threshing crew.

We children waited with eagerness for when we would be called to sit at the extended dining room table. We knew it would be filled with fried chicken, mashed potatoes and gravy, pumpkin pie, Jell-O with whipped cream (the real thing), deviled eggs, some kind of a green vegetable, tea or coffee for the adults, and chocolate milk for the children. Was it any wonder that after eating this meal, everyone wanted to take a nap?

Soon the large dinner was used up in our exercises. The adults would enjoy small talk and have a few moments of shut-eye. But we children, of course, wanted to play games outside. The girls played pom-pom-pull-away, hide-and-seek, and "London Bridge Is Falling Down"; and the boys played a game of softball.

This tradition began to die out when we children became teenagers. Who wanted to play those silly games? Who wanted to sit around and listen to the gossip of the adults?

When we teenagers moved into young adulthood, we had our own families to care for and new friends to see. The draw for dinner at Grandma's house disappeared.

It was sad to no longer see these families assembled around the extended dining room table. The fellowship that came from these dinners was deeply needed in our family. Of course, we did not realize it at the time. Today we look back and see how the tradition was so important.

Certain traditions are necessary in families and in the life of a nation. When my wife and I lived in China and Pakistan, we observed how certain traditions played a vital role in holding the tribes and nation together. In the United States we have lost this cohesion because our families no longer live in the same neighborhood in which we were born.

In China especially, the different seasons of the year were celebrated. The extended family gathered in a certain place to enjoy the fun and fellowship they all looked forward to. As we taught English classes in China, the students would tell us about these celebrations, like the New Moon Festival, the Lantern Festival, or certain meetings of their families. The students began planning how to get home because many of them lived many miles from their villages.

They did not celebrate Thanksgiving, for this is truly a United States festival, but they had other celebrations that far outdate ours. But much like our holiday gatherings, at their festivals food and drink were always the center of attraction with the time of meeting and visiting as a close second.

President Lincoln did our people a great favor in establishing a national Thanksgiving Day. This was especially true at the time of the Civil War. The nation needed a time of healing. From that time on, families enjoyed Thanksgiving dinner at Grandma's house for generations. Only as we have moved all over the nation has this tradition broken down. Our nation is missing out on a lot because of this lost tradition. Sure, some families do have the traditional dinner at Grandma's house, but there are not as many as there used to be.

Do you remember eating Thanksgiving dinner at Grandma's house? It was a real pleasure, and often I miss the times we assembled around the extended table. I can still hear the call, "Come to dinner!" We children would all rush to find our places at the table. Grace would be said, and the dishes of food would begin to travel from one hand to another…

Remember this tradition when that season arrives this year.

Men Marry Duplicates of Their Mothers

WHY DO MEN marry women who are duplicates of their mothers? Is it bred into them in the womb of their mother? Is it because this is the pattern they have had in their brain since birth? Is it genetic? Do men long for their mothers? Are they looking for an extension of the love found in their mothers?

Little boys will go outside to play and have fun for a few minutes and then return to their mothers. Apparently this gives them the assurance that their protector is still present. This lasts until about the age of six years. After this, boys still desire the protection of their mothers but not as frequently as they did in their younger years.

I see mothers as the protectors of the race. They will give their lives for their sons, if need be. Do men unconsciously sense this and marry a female for a companion who will take care of their offspring as their mother did?

As I think about my wife and mother, I see that they had and have many of the same characteristics. Mother, much like my wife, loved others and cherished each of her children. She was joyful most of the time, forgiving, unselfish, and tender. Both are and were devout believers in God and salvation through Jesus Christ. Both were and are unselfish in giving of themselves for the benefit of others.

However, there are also marked differences in the two women. My wife enjoys sexual relations. My mother put up with it. She had five children; my wife had three. Mom, until the time of change in her physical life, never knew when she would become pregnant again. Father was unwilling to use any protective measures. He wanted his rights no matter what took place. My wife and I took measures to see that we did not bring unwanted children into this world. My mother was about five feet tall and plump, even to the day she died. My spouse is about the same height, but slender. She weighs 109.5 pounds. Mom at one time weighed 180 pounds and in her later years probably weighed around 145 pounds.

There were also differences between my parents' relationship and my wife's and my relationship. Never in the eighteen years that I lived at home did I see my father take Mom in his arms and love her. My spouse and I daily love each other. We enjoy the touch of love.

The Bible says, "Leave your father and mother and become one with your wife."

Why do men marry women resembling their mothers? Why am I coming up with all questions and no apparent answers? Probably because I really never have read or heard the reason why men marry women like their mothers. (However, this thesis would make an excellent start for a doctoral dissertation.) If you have the answer to this question, please tell me.

On Family Leaving

TODAY OUR SON and his wife departed our place after a two-week visit. The four of us enjoyed each other, even though there is twenty-five years of difference in our ages. Even his wife seemed to enjoy being here. Of course, it helped that they had a separate place to sleep and a bit of privacy.

There is always a tug in my emotions when my children or grandchildren depart from my physical presence. Now that I am in my eighties, my children seem to mean much more to me than in the early years. It is a shame. My wife had the privilege of knowing them in a way that I never have and never will. Why? Because she was the vehicle through which they came to this planet. Oh, yes, I was responsible for impregnating her, but she was the one to carry them in her body and nurse each one. There is something about the mother that causes her children to have a special attachment to her. She is the one to whom they turn when pain of any type comes.

Memories flood in when the last bag is stowed in the trunk of the automobile, the "good-byes" have been said, and the hugs and kisses are over. Then each person wishes there were just a few more minutes to talk, one more hug to give, and an extra kiss to bestow. But time for such adventure is over; the driver of the car signals he is impatient to be on his way.

I have been such a driver. I also have experienced sadness in my emotions when the time came to depart from my loved ones. As the years piled up in my life, these times became very memorable. It would be wonderful to feel my mother's arms around me one more time or to see the look of happiness when I came to her home and ate a meal she had prepared. To her, I always looked thin, when in reality my weight was more than adequate.

This same sense came over me these past two weeks when our youngest son and his wife were with us. His mother did not do the cooking because he wanted to do it and did so. An excellent cook he is, even if his father says so. For the first time, I learned that he had intended to go to chef school when in fact he went to college and then into the US Air Force for three years. How little some of us fathers know about the plans of our offspring.

On a sad note, as I think of these times of family leaving, I remember how forty-one years ago my father-in-law helped me to back a travel trailer we were using out into the heavy traffic on the highway in front of his house. A week later, as we drove into our driveway at home in Nebraska, the telephone was ringing; we learned that he had died just a few days after we had departed. Our family had left my father-in-law's home, not knowing that we would never see him again on this earth.

When families leave each other, we are never assured that we shall meet again here in our earthly life. Each person believes he or she will see loved ones again here, but we have no assurance of such a meeting.

My wife and I know we shall see her father again because all of us believe in Jesus Christ and the resurrection. This truth is stamped in our souls. Grief has been assuaged by the sure knowledge of the resurrection of the soul and body at the last day.

The First Year of Marriage

DO YOU REMEMBER your first year of marriage? What was it like? Or perhaps you are not married but hope to be. Whatever the case, read on.

People speak of being "crazy in love." That would describe our first year of marriage. Neither of us could keep from being in contact with our spouse. We just had to be in each other's presence. Sure it was sexual attraction, but we also just wanted to be in the presence of the other person. It seemed as if we could never get enough of each other. If we could have crawled inside the other's body, we would have done so. To this day, there are times when I want to be as close to my wife of sixty-six years as possible. I want her to be closer than my skin.

In addition to wanting to be together, we were also very possessive of each other. Our dating had been over a one-and-a-half-year period while we were in college. The college would not allow couples to marry within the academic year, or we would not have waited that long. In the summer of 1942, after the academic year was completed, we traveled by the Wabash Railroad to Adrian, Michigan, where my wife was reared.

On the first day of June 1942, we walked down the aisle of her home church and before our families were married by my father, a pastor. It was a very simple ceremony. No music, almost like a Quaker wedding. My wife's sister was the bridesmaid, and my younger brother was my best man. At the chancel of the church, my father read the marriage service, and after prayer, we were pronounced husband and wife. Of course, we also had the traditional time of kissing before the families.

My wife's grandparents were deceased, but my grandfather was present, as were my paternal grandmother and her husband, my step-grandfather.

Outside the church, my wife's eldest half brother's wife took a picture of us, the only one we have of the wedding. Later, in the afternoon, after an excellent meal in my father-in-law's home, more pictures were taken. It was a hot June day, so we were in clothing that was as comfortable as possible.

Because we did not own a car, my father-in-law loaned us his, and we started on a three-day honeymoon over Lower Michigan. That evening we stayed in the best hotel I could afford, The Olds in Lansing, Michigan. We had a room on the tenth floor. I can still remember not signing in as husband and wife. The clerk had to remind me of the necessity. We all laughed about this beginning.

That evening we enjoyed each other to the fullest.

The next morning we began driving around portions of Michigan that we desired to see, ending in a small town in the central portion of the state. There my parents had invited many of our friends to a wedding shower; the room was full of those who had known me for years. A former female friend, whom I had dated for one-and-a-half-years, was present. Did she want to see who had captured me?

We stayed with my parents that evening. The next day we drove back to Adrian, returned the loaned car to my father-in-law, and caught the train back to our residence in Huntington, Indiana, arriving late in the evening. We found our way to the upstairs apartment we had rented and fell into bed.

On Monday I reported for work at an armament factory. I had been hired as a straw boss because of my deferment by the local draft board as a ministerial student. As a foolish young man, I had not told the foreman that I would be absent to get married. They inquired about where I had been. I informed them that I was now a married man. To this the foreman replied, "Why didn't you tell me? We would have given you leave to get married." Fortunately, they did not fire me, partially because it was difficult to find male employees.

As a young, married male, my mind was not on the job. I was working seven days a week and earning thirty-five dollars per week, which was big money for a young man who had been earning ten cents per hour at the college. My background of being reared in a denomination that was against war soon caused me to leave that position as the straw boss of a line of females.

Meanwhile, my wife was hired as the secretary to a denominational leader. But soon after, we found out she was pregnant with our first child, even though we had attempted to use the birth control methods of the time. Her workdays were over when she began to show her condition.

I went from one job to another, finally leaving college, returning to Michigan, and working as a janitor and bus driver in the local school system. After this, I went to work as a machine operator in a factory and returned to college.

Our first son was born in April of 1943. After that, my wife taught in a country school. That lasted a portion of a year, and then we moved to Kalamazoo, where I was in college, and she obtained a job in a pharmacy factory.

Looking back now, I wonder why my young wife stayed with her wandering husband. She would reply, "I loved him." This has been the story over the sixty-six years of our marriage. Once, after we were married, she told me, "The first day I saw you I knew I was going to marry you."

Children

LAST EVENING I talked with my daughter via the telephone. To me, she is still my child, even though she will be sixty-three years old on October 30. My wife, in turn, views her six foot, three inch son as her baby because he was the last child born. Why is it that we view our offspring as our children even though they are adults?

We often see the same sort of thing to our siblings. My daughter sees her six-feet-three-inch-tall brother as her "little" brother, even though he is sixty-one years old, married, and now a retired teacher. Maybe one of the reasons is because she took care of him when he was her "little" brother. She was a "little mother" to him and attempted to see that his wants were met.

What happens to us emotionally that causes us to internally attach certain titles to our offspring or family members?

In my family of origin, my eldest sister was thirty-eight months younger than I. I never felt attached to my brothers and sisters, even though intellectually I knew they were my blood relatives. To this day, I know they are from the same parents, but I seem a stranger in their homes. We are of the same blood, but we are very different from each other.

On the other hand, our three children seem very attached to each other. This has especially seemed true in their adult years. Perhaps because I was occupied in my work for seventy and eighty hours per week, I did not perceive or fully understand how closely they were attached to each other as children. Today, when they get together in our home at a holiday or in one of their homes, they seem to have real joy in being in the company of each other.

How wise God was in giving us children who in turn are a joy to each other! Oh, yes, I am aware that some families do not seem to enjoy the same attachment that our three children do.

As an eighty-six-year-old male, little children are a joy for me to see but not to handle or care for. This is the privilege of their parents or of other responsible adults. As a counselor I enjoy working with one small child at a time, not a group.

On the other hand, my wife is thrilled to be in the company of many little folks. She beams all over in their presence, and they beam back at her. There is an attachment that takes place automatically between my wife and a child or the children she meets. Somehow God has endowed her with a special talent for being with small children. She has something that comes from her inner personality. Children seem to feel safe with her and she with them.

Parents and adults have a huge responsibility when it comes to being in the presence of children. They watch our every move, sense our emotions, and respond accordingly.

Children are God's gift to the human race. How do you care for a child?

Easter and the Dinner

WHEN YOU SEE "Easter Dinner," what comes to mind? An abundance of food that is more than any ten people can eat? People and more people (at least this has been my experience)? When was the last time you were a part of such a gathering?

My family used to have such performances but no more. We all live far apart now. Our children are scattered over the nation. My brothers and sister are two thousand miles away.

My wife's family, on the other hand, lives 125 miles away. We attend such gathering with them on Easter and Thanksgiving. They enjoy such gatherings, when old times and places familiar to all can be remembered. Usually, one of the main topics discussed is how the city where they all lived has changed. This street is now wider, such and such bridge is being rebuilt...and this is all taking place while people are "feeding their faces."

My part of the gathering is to listen to the family and friends talk and to learn; thus, when my wife asks me a question after these gatherings, I at least seem to have some knowledge about the conversation. My listening helps me save face with my wife. Of course, these activities are meaningless to me, but at least I can seem to have been awake. Who would not be when food is in abundance?

Long ago, my family enjoyed such affairs. Fond memories register in my thinking of these times. Pictures still resonate in my mind as I remember the events that took place each year. Usually we gathered in the home of my maternal grandmother or of some of the close family. Living in Michigan, families were close to each other since the state is only 200 miles in length and 150 miles in width. These gatherings would find aunts, uncles, and children all over the place, eating and laughing as the events of the present and past were recalled.

Did your family have such gatherings? Midwestern families seemed to revel in these affairs. Gatherings such as ours were common in the extended families all around us. These gatherings afforded the families the opportunity to keep in touch, see the new babies, and listen to the latest gossip. Often church and politics were the main discussions of the men; babies and marriages were the topics for the women. Children romped and played all sorts of games, and everyone came away from the day exhausted but happy.

Children in this generation do not realize what they are missing in not knowing their cousins, aunts, and uncles. The extended family was very real to a person after these meetings. The families today, because we are living all over the USA, do not have the opportunity to enjoy these privileges.

There are some exceptions, however. For example, where my wife and I reside, there is a large population of Hispanics. They fill the parks to overflowing each and every Sunday and overflow the same parks on festive occasions. Each family seems to have a certain area they have claimed as their own.

Many of these families live in very cramped circumstances; thus, the parks afford them the opportunity to be in the open and allow the children to romp and play their games.

During Easter, more properly titled Resurrection Sunday, what is your favorite memory? Why not take time to recall it today? Your life may be much richer if you do.

Section Three

Community Life

The Volunteer

HAVE YOU EVER enjoyed volunteering? If you have, you know what a joy it is to help others. My wife and I volunteer each week at a local hospital. For four hours she works in the gift shop and I answer questions at the information desk.

In her job, my wife helps to keep an eye on those who decide to take an object without paying for it—in other words, those who are stealing. My job is to answer questions for folks who come in to see patients or to help those who have been patients. Generally the questions asked are the following: "Where is the ICU?" "Where is the surgical waiting room?" "Where do I pay my bill?" "Is the restaurant open?" "Where is the emergency room?" And the list goes on and on.

These positions require a person to enjoy interaction with others. Usually people are gracious and kind; only on rare occasions does one meet a difficult individual. In cases such as these, if it is impossible for me to help the difficult person, I phone the security staff and they come at once to assist in quieting the individual.

Because this hospital was once known as "the country hospital," people still think of it as such. However, this is no longer true. Today this hospital is part of the University Medical Center and has doctors seeing patients who in past years would have been in the University system. Currently, the hospital has over three hundred doctors seeing patients in the clinics attached to it.

Stories are told each day that I work as a volunteer at the information desk. Often people just need an ear to hear their stories. These people are helped by a sympathetic listener being behind the desk. It is my belief that most humans need a sympathetic ear to listen to their desires and longings. We serve God and our fellowmen when we lend a listening ear.

Thus far in this article I have focused only on what my wife and I do. What about other volunteers? What positions do they fill in this hospital? One volunteer we know pushes a cart with magazines and books she gives to patients who are confined to a bed. Also, she lends a listening ear.

Another volunteer I know and see in the hospital is a chaplain. He was in the service for twenty years. After retiring, he served in the local VA hospital until a new head chaplain came and decided his help was not needed. Now he is active three and four days a week as a chaplain in this hospital. In his early years he desired to be a minister, but his family did not view this occupation as one they wanted to live with. Now, all alone, he is able to serve where he feels God is calling him.

Today, the younger generation is not volunteering as mine did. Once we were known as the volunteering nation of the world, but this is no longer so. Now other nations have people who are beginning to volunteer in their country. Some are even going to other countries to volunteer.

Among those who are volunteering in our country and around the world, people from religious groups are in the forefront. Over many generations the church has supplied different personnel to meet the needs of religious, educational, and medical services. Presently, some are helping nations to drill wells, bringing in fresh, pure water for the people. This aid has cut down on the disease problems that were so prevalent in nations with limited funds to meet such health needs. Others are helping to bring education to nations who have had very limited teachers to meet the educational standards of the world.

Teachers and educators are needed all over the world right now. My wife and I know this to be true from personal experience. We volunteered for a year to teach English as a second language in a remote area of China. Then, after our return from China, our church asked us to volunteer on a short-term basis to help meet the needs of a large school in Pakistan. Worldwide the need is huge, as evident by the advertisements in magazines asking for such personnel.

Your life will be very meaningful when you see the need and fulfill it as a volunteer. I challenge you to look into serving as a short-term volunteer. You will know fulfillment if you do this.

Volunteer today!

Chinese Friends

OUR SIX-MONTH TOUR of teaching English as a second language was about to expire when she walked into our apartment on the bottom floor of the building. She was very young, just in her first year or two of a college career. After giving us her Chinese name, she said, "My English name is Jackie. The last foreign teacher said my name sounded like that." Jackie had been appointed our translator. She was to be our go-between, translating from Mandarin to English and vice versa. Jackie became our constant companion, that is, when she could; classes were in her way, plus eating, sleeping, and washing clothes.

When we found out we were to be shuffled around from one place to another, our enjoyment ceased. For one thing, Hubei University did not believe we could do the work that needed to be done; thus, we had been sent into the mountains, where we were listed under Shiyan University, but we would actually be teaching Second Automotive Works. Shiyan University did not have the funds to pay us, but the institute desired an older couple, especially since I had a doctorate. In 1986 China had few teachers with doctoral degrees.

Still, Jackie was to be our guide and helper wherever we went in the city of Wuhan or anywhere else in China. She was one of the outstanding students in the Foreign Language Department of Hubei University. This school had been a teacher's college turning out teachers, whether they desired to be teachers or not. China then had the policy of looking over the national academic needs and placing students where they wanted them. All this has changed today. Now students can choose the career in which they desire to be trained, but back then the central government chose your profession. If the nation needed more doctors, you might find yourself sent to medical school. If the nation needed more bodies to fill slots in the governmental structure, you went and did not outwardly complain.

Because the school was very poor, at the bottom of the academic scale, eight students slept in one room, and they could have only four showers a month. After Jackie came to know us much better, one day when it was very cold she asked, "May I use your bathtub?" Of course we responded in the affirmative, and as long as we were there she would use our bathtub as needed. She was our friend, and we were her friends.

Much later on she wrote the top exam to qualify for the opportunity to earn her doctorate in educational psychology at the University of New South Wales in Australia. A male student and Jackie ranked as numbers one and two at the top of the exam. The heads of the university were determined to give the scholarship to the male student; however, the former president of Hubei said, "No, this woman has the top score on the exam, and she should be granted the scholarship." Thus, Jackie was off to her doctoral studies in Australia.

Jackie completed four years in that university and graduated with her PhD. She was married by then, and fortunately her husband and her baby daughter were able to live with her in Sydney, Australia. Her husband had his master's degree, making him better educated than many Australians. He found work as an orderly in a hospital, but he never enjoyed the people of Australia. Perhaps, just perhaps, they showed racial discrimination toward this Chinese person.

Three years ago we visited Jackie and her family in Wuhan, where she is now the department Chairwoman of foreign languages. Under the one-child law, the little girl born to this couple is their only offspring. She was and is a very intelligent child who has a flair for the designing of women's clothes. She hopes to be known for that ability someday. Presently, she is in senior high school. She is the beloved child of her father, however, he does not allow her to run the family as some let their little boys do.

Our lives have been blessed because of the way in which God worked to change us from one college to another, even though we did not really like going to one of the "furnace cities" of China. Wuhan is extremely hot and humid in the summer. Everyone who can leaves as often as they are able, going to a cooler climate or to the ocean side.

Jackie is our friend to this day. By e-mail today, I received pictures taken of her family on a recent vacation. Now fifty years old, Jackie is no longer the slender female we met when she came to our apartment to escort us to Wuhan University. Years have made a difference in her physical beauty. To begin with, she was a plain person; but soon her personality showed forth, and it still does. May her daughter follow in her mother's footsteps.

The VA Hospital

HAVE YOU EVER needed to use the VA hospital? Currently, the Veterans Administration hospital system is under intense scrutiny. From the news I've heard over the radio and television, the vets returning from the Iraq War are not receiving the medical care they need. The head personnel are being fired, and a commission has been set up to look into the circumstances. Is this all that will take place? Will the care needed for these men and women change for the better? Commissions only report findings; it takes action on the part of Congress to change the treatment of vets.

Only this morning I was in the local VA hospital. My appointment was kept almost on time, and the MD, whom I have seen before, took care of me in a professional fashion.

My care in this local facility has been excellent. The internist that serves me is listed as one of the two hundred best doctors in the city of Tucson. She does everything possible to see that my physical needs are met medically. Her attitude is, "I am here to serve you. What is your need today?" Really, the medical team as a whole has been the best. Of course, my needs have not been mental but mostly those of a body that is wearing out. After eighty-six years of service, what can I expect from my body?

The nurses I have had the good fortune to know have been caring people. They are in nursing because they want to help people. Generally they do not make a large income. A few doing special needs do, but most only make a good living, nothing special.

My spouse and I have three nieces who are nurses; two are NPs, and one is a burn specialist (she spent twenty years in the army in this occupation). One of the NPs stayed in the army and obtained the rank of colonel. She retired and immediately stepped into a position where she earned seventy dollars per hour in a private clinic. In making this type of wage, she is the exception to the rule.

The medical facilities at the VA hospital are some of the best I have used in my years of medical needs. Of course, they probably should be when you think of the millions of dollars spent on these operations.

In addition to the VA hospital, the city of Tucson has several excellent hospitals, including the University of Arizona Medical School. One of the reasons my spouse and I moved to Tucson was to have excellent medical care. In the city where we resided for eight years, there was only one hospital, and it was controlled by the medical establishment. Today, nine years later, there are two hospitals, plus a hospital for the mentally ill. Of course, the city now has a population of over one hundred thousand. When we lived there, the population was not quite seventy-five thousand with twenty thousand of those being students in the local four-year college.

One thing I like about the VA hospital is that personnel attempt to take care of crucial needs the very day the veteran calls. This is better than what most medical offices are able to do. Usually patients wait for several days before they can be seen. This is one reason there are so many emergency offices in the city. In these facilities a patient is seen as soon as possible on the day the need is made known. This is as it should be.

What is your experience with the VA, or do you have any experience at all? Veterans of my age are dying at the rate of fourteen hundred each day. Soon the needs for the VA hospital will have all but vanished. The Second World War vets, Korean War vets, and those from other small wars we have engaged in will be gone. What will the situation be then? If we hit real economic difficulties, how will the federal government fund the many medical facilities over the nation? This question has yet to be answered.

Today

TODAY I SAW beauty in all of its fullness. A mother with twins came into the hospital waiting room. The two, a girl and a boy, were adorable. A certain luster in the eyes of the one-year-old girl set her apart. The innocence of a baby is heartwarming.

The little boy was all boy. What do I mean? He was moving all the time and especially interested in his bottle. Have you ever witnessed a little boy who wants to eat *now*?

These twins had individual carriages. Grandma was present, and you could see that she delighted in the children. Even though she could not speak English, she was able to express her fondness for these two. Language, other than the spoken word, is very effective. The smile on her face each time she looked at the babies, the tenderness with which she spoke to them in Spanish, and the soft caress of her hands on each child sent a message of fond excitement to each little one.

One could tell the babies were well developed mentally, physically, and emotionally. They were very alert, their eyes sparkled, the motions of their hands were smooth, and the understanding showing in their faces told me that these were children well on their way to being quality individuals.

I wondered what their seven-year-old sister must have thought when the two new babies came to take her place. Did she accept them joyfully, or was their hatred on her part for someone else taking her coveted first place? Did she view them as dolls to be played with? Was she Mother's little helper? All of these are possibilities. But not having the privilege of knowing the seven-year-old sister, I have no way of seeing the dynamics in the family. If big sister is a normal child, there probably is jealousy over these babies taking up all their mother's time. Big sister gets what's left.

Some jealous children have attempted to kill the new arrivals. Parents have found the older sibling attempting to smother the new siblings. Hatred is strong when an only child is suddenly displaced. When the king or queen is pushed off the throne, tragedy may occur.

Children can be little monsters or little angels. How the parents inform the older children of the coming of a new family member is a key to the integration of the new member. Parents have the key to unlock the door of success or failure for the incoming babies and their siblings.

Two Old Ladies

ONE DAY AS I sat at the information desk, two old ladies took chairs by a window in the main lobby of the hospital. At first I did not pay any attention to them, but soon I could not help but pay attention, for one of the ladies proceeded to talk, talk, talk for two hours. The other lady just sat there and listened, occasionally saying yes or some other word, which just sent the first woman on a rampage with another harangue for at least a half hour.

These two women spent the afternoon seated by the window, doing nothing but talking. My thought was, *Doesn't the nonstop talker have anyone else to listen to her? Did she infringe upon the other lady, or were both of them starved for company?*

These questions set me to thinking, *How many old folks are starved for someone to listen to them?* Humans are made to communicate with each other. We have a built-in need to converse. This is one reason it is very good for retired elderly people to have animals to talk to. Some of the animals seem to understand what their elderly masters are saying, or at least they act as if they do. People who spend hours working with the elderly have found that these people live longer and are happier when they have a cat, dog, or bird to care for and talk to.

Is this why God created mankind? Let's look at what we know of God. Really all that we humans know about God is from what the great prophets and seers have recorded about God (in the Bible) and what we see in creation (Ps. 119; Rom. 1:20). We know that God has always been and that there are three persons in the Godhead, so they have always had each other to converse with. We have a picture of God the Father in the person of Jesus Christ. He told His disciples, "If you have seen me, you have seen the Father." So the picture we have of the Father is what we have recorded by the first-century people who spent three years with Jesus Christ and who by the turn of the first century had written down their observations and thoughts and what they remembered from what Christ taught them. This is what we have recorded in the New Testament. In these accounts, we see that Jesus Christ seemed to enjoy being with His followers. We certainly do not have everything He said and did written down, but we do have enough to get a glimpse of who God is, especially as the Father and lover of His creatures.

Genesis 1 records God saying, "Let us make man in our image and likeness" (v. 6). Mankind at his best is a small picture of God, for this is what God created. In making us in His image and likeness, He gave us a free will. I wonder if He ever regretted this act. Apparently God has a free will to do as He pleases, for we are made like Him. This free will places a huge responsibility upon our maker and the made, mankind. How we can use this free will is awesome.

The two old ladies were using their free will to talk. Maybe it was good, or perhaps not for those who are close to them. However, they seemed to be enjoying the use of what the Creator had bestowed upon them: talk, talk, talk, and more of the same.

Are not the created called upon to use what God gave them in an honorable and upright manner? I cannot say that the two old ladies were not doing so, but they certainly wore me out. Finally, they decided the time had come to leave, and as abruptly as they had begun, they departed the main lobby of the hospital. A deadly silence came over the place.

Friends

TODAY WE ARE sending in the mail a couple of books that we hope will help our friend in China who is rearing a teenage daughter. Some will say to me, "Why are you doing this?" My answer is "She is our friend." When we lived in China for a year, we got to know her. Over the years we have corresponded by e-mail. She has changed from a young lady to a married woman and the mother of one child, her daughter.

We have been blessed with many friends from around the world. We have friends in Wales, Pakistan, China, Japan, Mexico, Australia, and Costa Rica. Blessings have come to us as we have been given the privilege of knowing folks in these countries. And all this has happened in the last twenty years. My spouse and I never thought we would have the joy of traveling to, and making friends in, these different areas. But I am grateful that we have because our lives have been blessed through these friendships.

How do you describe a friend? Did you ever stop to think about how different your friends are from each other? As I think of our friends, some are close and very dear to us, while others are friends but not close. Each of these friends has a special place in our hearts. We still remember them for what they mean to us, and we hope that we mean something to them. Each of us has learned from the other person—from the person's customs, habits of life, and the traditions that go with the different countries in which they life. No person or country is the same. Even within a country the people we know are different from each other. Here in the United States we have friends who are Republicans and Democrats. Some of our friends have different religious backgrounds—Roman Catholic, Lutheran, Methodist, Southern Baptist, and Presbyterian. Each person has some particular characteristic, setting him or her apart from our other friends, and they all enrich our lives in some manner.

Friends are special gifts from God. They come into your life at a particular time and for a definite reason. The reason may have been fulfilled, but they are still your friends, some exceedingly close and other friends far away.

My daughter-in-law is my friend because she is married to my youngest son. We have a person in common. From this relationship, enjoyment has come. Further because we both write, she professionally and I as an aspiring author of fiction, we have a bond of friendship.

Who do you count as your friend or friends? Why not stop whatever you are doing and count the true friends you have? It is reported that if you have five close friends, you are a most fortunate person. Close friends are those persons you can tell anything to, no matter how horrid, and they continue as true friends. These persons should be valued as if they were made of gold with diamond crowns.

Friends, at one time we had many. As the years have sneaked up on us, the number of close friends has diminished. Age and death take those you can count as true friends. Of course, there are always friends on the fringes, but you do not tell them the gritty things that come into your life.

If you have five close friends, you are a most fortunate person. Keep them close to your bosom. They share the values you cling to.

Conversations in a Beauty Parlor

WHAT GOSSIP HAVE you heard in a beauty parlor? My friend, who is a beautician, tells me that women can hardly wait until they are seated in the chair before they begin to unload.

One day as I was having a haircut, a beautician was unloading on a client. It went something like this: "I don't care if he is out of a job; he still owes me my alimony check each month. That is what he was ordered to pay by the court. He left me to marry a younger woman. His responsibility is to do what the court ordered. Let him suffer as I did when he divorced me to marry her." This discourse went on for a period of time.

All people have the need to confide in other people. It seems to be the makeup of the human being. Do we feel better emotionally when we do this? Women will disclose the innermost secrets of their personal lives while in the chair. It is almost as if the person is in the confessional booth. They seem to have an inner need to tell all. If they would only do this when in a counseling session, it would not be necessary for them to tell all to the beautician. Perhaps the person doing the unloading feels safer with the lady behind the chair. Is it that they do not trust the pastor or counselor with their secrets?

Salt and Pepper

Older women seem to need to talk about their children and grandchildren. They delight in sharing the activities of both groups. Most older folks have children, grandchildren, and great-grandchildren. This gives the client plenty of ammunition to share with the beautician.

Often I wonder if the beautician wishes these ladies would keep their innermost secrets to themselves. I wonder, *Does the beautician need to wash her mind of what she has heard at the end of a busy day? Does the beautician keep a diary of what takes place as she works behind the chair?* If so, she will have plenty of information to share if she ever writes a book.

My older sister was a beautician. I need to ask her if she kept a diary of the conversations that took place when she had her shop.

On my part, it seems as if I relax once seated in the chair. A sense of peace comes over me. In this relaxed mode, you have to be careful of what you say. The room has many ears, not all of them closed.

It is not only in the beauty shop where we need to keep close tabs on what we allow to escape from our mouths. Other rooms have many ears also. This is especially true in a restaurant. We human beings become very talkative when food is present. Often if you listen closely, over the noise of the music, conversation, and the coming and going of the waiters, very salient information is divulged.

No doubt in this election year, much information is being passed between persons as they sit in restaurant booths. We US citizens feel that it is our privilege to speak out when the candidates are spending huge sums of money to win our votes.

Would it not be true in the beautician's chair that all the specialist would need to do is answer with "umm" a few times, and the person in the chair would just ramble on?

What have you heard as you were comfortably seated in a chair?

My Next-Door Neighbor

DO YOU HAVE a next-door neighbor? If you live in a village or city, usually you do. In a large city there are multiple neighbors. Unless you live on the ground floor, they are probably beside, below, and above you.

We live in a gated community. It is small when compared to other such communities; in all, there are ninety-eight residents. We have neighbors beside us and across from us. And over our back fence is a mobile home community with over eighteen hundred living areas. This group has been in existence for over twenty-five years. They were out in this area when all you could hear were the wild animals native to the desert.

My next-door neighbor purchased his patio home three years ago after the ninety-year-old lady who lived there died and her son didn't want the property. My neighbor is of medium stature and addicted to cigarettes. He is rarely in the house. But when he is living there, apparently he enjoys being by himself. He does not take part in the operation of the community and never appears at the community meetings, not even the annual meeting, but he is friendly when we meet.

About the time he purchased the property, our neighbor married a lady from Sierra Vista. She has a home and a business in that city. This was his third marriage.

Our neighbor's second wife and their daughter live in the Detroit, Michigan, area. Every so often he flies back to see his daughter, and on an occasion she has spent time with him in the summer here in Arizona.

This past year our neighbor flew a fighter plane to Thailand. He spent many hours in the cockpit, and the plane was gassed up from a tanker plane while in the air. As I have seen this operation on TV, it looks to me as if this is a very "tricky" bit of craftsmanship. How the tanker with its long gasoline boom can maneuver into the tiny filler on the speeding plane is truly amazing.

The other day a "for sale" sign was posted in front of our neighbor's home. He is selling it and plans to build a new home in Sierra Vista. He, a lieutenant colonel, is currently on furlough from American Airlines, where he has been a pilot for many years. He will retire in two more years and make his residence with his wife in Sierra Vista. I guess he will need to find some other attraction to keep him occupied besides flying. Who knows?

One day we heard a lot of noise outside his home. Looking out, I saw a man with a ladder about to scale the wall. He climbed the ladder and inspected the roof and structure. Later, the real estate agent, a woman, was here with two men. The men went up on the roof and inspected it (I presume). Then another man inspected the interior of the house with the agent. Since that day, nothing more has been seen of the agent or the presumed buyer.

It's interesting how "nosy" we have been. Because there is only a twelve-inch wall between his home and mine, I am interested in who purchases that home. Because of the heavy insulation in the walls and a three-inch gap between them, very little noise comes through. Still, I am interested in who will occupy the home next door.

How about your next-door neighbor? Do you hear the music and programs coming from his or her sound system or television? Living as we do in cities, very close together, noise is a very important factor to each homeowner.

Do you know your next-door neighbors? Do you enjoy their company?

Ladies Aid Society

DID YOU EVER hear of the Ladies Aid Society? These groups of women perform many works to help our national life, for example, earning money to help local churches.

There are other groups that have different names for the same type of organization. Many of these organizations are in the process of finding ways and means to assist in funding the programs they wish to see created to help members of the public. For example, some groups of like nature assist mental health organizations in earning money to fund programs that help people who do not have the money to pay for the therapy.

The Ladies Aid Society, I remember, was affiliated with the church in which my father was a pastor. This group was primarily devoted to raising money to take care of different projects in the local congregation. Sometimes they even had bake sales to help pay the preacher's small salary.

Some other women in our congregation belonged to the Missionary Society. This group raised money to provide the means whereby the missionaries overseas could continue their work. A tug-of-war would take place in the congregation as to which group would have first honors for doing the most rewarding work. It was distressing for the pastor, who wanted to see both groups make progress.

Generally, the Ladies Aid Society would meet for an evening meal in a farm home. We teenagers enjoyed such meetings because it was possible for us to enjoy many of the delicious foods that the farm wives would cook. Perhaps you remember your teen years when, except for girls, food was the primary thought on your mind. We visualized both as delicious.

My paternal grandmother is part of my earliest memories because she took me to these women's meetings. There I was passed around, and each elderly woman had to hold me and plant a juicy kiss on my cheek. As a baby I could not resist, but in my later toddler years I expressed strong objections, especially to the juicy, wet kisses from the old grandmas.

Did you ever attend a Ladies Aid Society meeting? Such meetings were the spice of life for a toddler and, especially if young females were present, for teenage boys. When we were teenagers, the young females always caused us "guys" to pay special attention. If the sponsor of a meeting wanted young males to attend, all that person needed to advertise was that a young lady would be present. Even if it wasn't advertised, somehow the males seemed to be able to find out who would be present—good-bye food, welcome females!

To this day, I fondly remember these meetings with the food, the girls, and all. While the women were holding their meeting inside the house, we young folk were outside playing whatever games were in vogue at the time. Since such meetings took place in the years of the Depression, very little entertainment was offered outside the home because we had no extra money to spend on a good time. So we just made do with the games long familiar to us. It is strange how quickly young people, when forced to find responsible recreation, can create their own enjoyment—no game boards, just fun doing anything.

Women's Missionary Society

WOMEN MAKE THE world go round, especially through works of charity. When I was four years old, my grandmother, a pastor, took me to an afternoon meeting of this women's group. Grandmother was a powerhouse as far as missionary work was concerned. She had been a missionary in Canada for her denomination in the early twentieth century.

My father would tell of the denominational executives coming to their home on the planes of Alberta, Canada. It was a grand time for the adults and a small child. Old friends from those years were still in power within Grandmother's denomination. She had close ties with these leaders. Thus, my grandmother could talk with them and feel completely at home in their presence. And when grandmother, as a pastor, spoke to the women in the missionary group, she had authority, for she knew these men and women personally. When she spoke of such folk, it was a personal matter. They were real flesh and bones. This small denomination knew these leaders.

When staying with my grandmother on the farm where she lived with her second husband (my natural grandfather had died some years earlier in an accident), I was expected to go along with her to these meetings. Thus, early in my life, being with women in meetings came naturally. Later on as a pastor and still later in my career when I was working primarily as a counselor, working with women did not give me pause.

For me as a child, these meetings were always interesting in two ways: 1) Early on I learned facts about missions and the personnel who carried on the work, both at home and overseas. 2) Food was always present, sweets especially, and what child does not enjoy sweets? The women always tried out their favorite pie and cake recipes at the gatherings. I can still hear them exclaiming, "My, this is good! But I had better not eat too much; I need to watch my weight." Then they would proceed to have two pieces of cake or a large helping of a favorite pie, plus coffee or tea.

In contrast to the parts of the meetings I enjoyed, an action which revolted me as a small child was being passed around to the women and being kissed by each one. Sometimes the perfume was just too much. I would wiggle and attempt to get free, but Grandmother would see that each woman had her turn to love on her small grandson. Needless to say, I was the "apple of her eye."

In my mind's eye, those farmhouse moments still loom large. A driveway would lead to the garage. Beside the garage would be a large, white frame house. This house would have a rear door, where most people would enter, and a front door for special occasions. The front door was used for the pastor to call on the family or for the women coming to the meeting to enter; otherwise on a weekday without fanfare you entered by the rear door.

Usually a farm dog lay close by or a collection of cats attempting to rush through the door to have something to eat. Often over the rear door, a cover had been erected, where the farm members would remove their muddy shoes and hang up their coats and hats. When a friend came by during the week, this formality was dispensed with. He or she would enter and then, if it was wintertime, remove the muddy footwear, coats, and hats.

After I had eaten my pie or cake and had a glass of water or milk and the women had passed me around to be kissed, Grandmother would allow me to go outside to play while the meeting took place inside the house. If the dog was friendly, we would have fun chasing each other. If not, the cats and I would make friends. Of course, if other women brought their children to the meetings, then it was an exceptionally fun time. We would play hide-and-seek, pom-pom-pull-away, and any running games that would use up our pie- or cake-induced energy.

Finally we—the exhausted, sweaty children—would wear out and hope that there was a large tree under which we could rest. Usually by this time the meeting was over, our rides would arrive, and we would be on our way home.

Memories of the Women's Missionary Society meetings are fond to envision. Whether my memory is completely correct or not, well, you take the story from there.

Section Four

The Modern Age

Computer Frustration

DOES COMPUTER FRUSTRATION ever consume you? At this very moment it has me in its grip. It would appear that I am still at the typewriter stage of writing. Operating these machines takes an engineer, a computer engineer.

My friends say it is very simple—yes, for them but not for me. It all seems so simple to my friend. Of course, he has taught it for many years, and he is a bit younger than I. My retention rate seems to be going downhill rapidly. Everything I do on this machine has to be drummed into my head again and again. The simple process of transferring an item I get on the Internet becomes complicated to me when I want to send it on to another party. My friends and brother-in-law send all manner of items to me. It's second nature to them—how come I am so dumb?

Like I said, it is necessary for me to do the same procedure over and over and over before it settles into my gray matter. Could it be that age has anything to do with this imprinting process? Tuesday, while at the information desk in the hospital, a fifty-year-old woman, who is now attending the University of Arizona, told me she was having problems with retention. She appeared to be a very intelligent individual. So perhaps I am not the only one who, after the age of six, has retention problems.

Salt and Pepper

My writing on a subject every day is an attempt on my part to keep my retrieval processes in shape. One day it appears they are working quite well, and the next day it seems as if all I learned the previous day has flown away on the "red eye" express. It is disgusting to have this happen; also, it tells me my eighty-six years of age are catching up with my mental processes.

Today while volunteering as the hospital chaplain on the fourth floor, I came upon a female patient who was "down in the dumps." She was ill not only physically but also mentally. It was not within my professional privilege to inquire very deeply as to why she was in this condition; but after leaving that room, I wondered what situation was causing her depression.

Computer frustration is something like this young female patient: she did not know exactly what to do. This is the situation in which I find myself. Which way do I go now?

My publisher has sent me the hard and soft covers for the fictional story I wrote about Legion, whom Jesus healed of demon possession. Somehow in my attempt to get the material up and on its way over the Net, I lost what the publisher sent me. Now what should I do? Call Xlibris, my publisher, and tell them of my mistake, or ask them what they suggest I do about my computer acting as it does? They could care less about my computer and its antics or me and my mistakes. What they want me to do is look over the e-mail and tell them whether it is OK.

The computer mess causes me to wonder if it is worth the effort to publish my story; however, with $900 sunk in the project, it is not something I want to back out of. Tomorrow I will call the cover design manager and tell him of my need to have the cover design sent again over the Internet.

Tell me how fifty-six thousand books are published each year with only a fraction of them making it on to the bookshelves of bookstores and the discount houses. I'm pleased that my income is not predicated upon my book being sold by the millions. However, there are those souls who make a decent living doing that.

The Big Box Store

AREAS OF OUR country are passing measures to keep the large, factory-like buildings where the buyer can have all his or her needs met under one roof out of their borders. Do you have such a store in your community? We are looking at one of these stores being built locally as soon as the county gets the roadwork done to allow the traffic flow necessary to support such a store. If all goes well, beginning the first of July, the total package will come together, and we shall have this type of store under construction.

Although I am not from Missouri, the saying "I'll believe it when I see it" is my motto. This area of the county has been promised such enjoyment before, but the powers that be have not produced. Why has this not occurred? Small merchants have fought it, and the politicians who represent this area have listened to the small merchants, and the store has been kept out. Certain citizens who are against this sign of progress or who have not seen the building of the big box store as a sign of progress have used their power to keep the local merchants happy.

Most of the citizens in our area of the county would enjoy having their needs met in one place. This type of store is supposed to meet these needs. Also, the stores advertise the large number of people who will be employed if the store is built. Small merchants say this is not true, for they employ more people than the big box store will. True, over the whole of our nation, the small businesspeople or companies do have larger numbers of employees. But as to this area of the county, there is no other large employer. All the businesses employ only a few people per establishment. What they are saying under a different guise is "The big box store will run us out of business. We cannot compete with their large purchasing power."

As for consumers, most could care less about the small businessman being out of business. What they are looking for is the best buy for the dollar. The big box store seems to have the answer. A person looks at the cost of an item in the large store and at the same item in the small business. He or she often finds that the needed item can be purchased for less money in the large store because of the ability of the big box store to purchase the product needed at a reduced price per item.

The average person does not seem to care where he or she spends his or her money if he or she can obtain more for the money spent in the larger store, which is controlled from some area outside the local confines. The Republican Party seems to support this concept, whereas the Democrat Party supports the opposite concept. It will be interesting to see what will happen with the presidential elections taking place. With employment at an all-time high, the "ins" will say that they caused this to happen and the "outs" will say, "Give us a chance; we can do even better."

From what I have read, an unemployment rate of 4.5 percent is about as low as our nation can go with the major factors of old age creeping up on our employees, job discrimination in vogue, and illnesses of different origins all making it very difficult to lower this figure. When I read of nations having an unemployment rate of 10 to 20 percent, it looks to me as if the USA is doing very well.

Currently there are signs of the unemployment rate rising. Motor car companies are laying off employees, house building is down 17 percent, and large inventories in factories are making companies think twice before adding employees. Interest rates have been juggled around in all factors of our money market; thus, purchasers are not sure where to look for the money they need. Our nation is over its head in credit card debt, and this, in turn, makes it impossible for a person or family to further go into debt to purchase items they believe they need. Last I read, the average family owes more than five thousand dollars on their credit cards.

In addition, the national government, to finance an unpopular war, is now in trillions of dollars of debt. If China, Japan, and England decide not to purchase any more of our bonds, we are in deep trouble as a nation, and our treasury is defunct. Our nation and the total world will fall into a worldwide depression, making the 1929 year look as if we were rich. If this should occur, we could do no less than forgo paying the interest on the bonds, and our national name as the richest nation in the world would fall into the ditch of the unreliable money people. After World War II, Germany, under their chancellor, had to do this very thing. This is what placed their government back on a firm financial footing. We may be forced to do the same. There is no way this debt can be paid off under present circumstances. A rich nation can become an impoverished nation almost overnight under foolish management.

Will this nation, known as the richest nation in the world, be forced to do what the economists in Germany had to do to bring our economy back to a healthy state? This may happen very soon; only time will tell. Let us hope that those who control the money supply of the USA exercise wisdom in their decisions.

Cell Phones 1

CELL PHONES ARE all over the world.

In China they are taking the place of conventional telephone service. As you walk down the street, it seems as if each and every pedestrian has a cell phone and its service. They rent out the phone for a certain amount of money and time. This saves users the price of a phone, yet they can still be connected to the known world.

The expansion of cell phone service over the world has changed the total concept of being connected in any place one may travel. You can now use a cell phone when doing business all around the world or for a friendly call to a loved one a continent away.

Do you imagine that the inventors of the cell phone ever envisioned the way the little phone would conquer the world in the field of communications? With strong competition from many companies, the growth of cell phone service has jumped beyond their fondest expectations.

With the competition from different companies, companies are adding new services in hopes that users will drop their company and move to what the consumer believes is a better quality of service. In situations such as these, what the user needs to do is look into the fine points of the contract that the company demands the user sign. Often the first reading of the blurb from the company does not stand up in the light of day. The companies have their best lawyers write these contracts, giving the company all the rights; the user is the loser.

The next time you decide another company will meet your demands more accurately, read the fine print; don't listen to the pitch the salesperson gives you. These companies impose heavy fines if you leave them before the end of the contract that most of them ask you to sign. I repeat: *read the fine print before you sign a cell phone contract.*

At times I see a person in rags with a cell phone to his or her ear. How do folks like these intend to pay for the service? Perhaps they do not intend to pay for the service. Sometimes it is difficult to catch up with these drifters. They move very quickly from place to place and from city to city. Even within cities they are experts at keeping out of the hands of the law or collection agencies. Collection agencies are only for operating against honest people.

This past week my phone stopped working. It had been in use for two years, but this summer my sister's puppy chewed it up, at least the cover and the antenna. Both were replaced, but it has not performed well ever since. Recently it decided to stop all together. I called T-Mobile, and the young lady on the other end of the line was most helpful in attempting to make my phone work again but with no success. Finally she said, "I think your battery is gone." She gave me the name of a local dealer that could help. Well, he couldn't, but he did send me to a company that had what I needed, a new battery. The young woman behind the counter installed the new battery, and now the phone is as good as new.

The magic of cell phones never stops amazing me. With no telephone line connected to my phone, when I dial a number, that signal goes to a tower some distance away, and from that tower it goes to others across the country until it reaches the destination I have dialed on my phone. Almost like magic but not quite. Electronic signals go out over the airwaves, and each tower picks up the signal until it reaches the proper location.

Cell Phones 1

As I travel across the country, I see towers all over the landscape. Lights are blinking at the top of the towers to ensure safety for air traffic, and also to keep the towers from being destroyed. I can sit in my comfortable chair and dial the number of my daughter in a small Iowa town. My son does volunteer work and moves about, but he has a cell phone, and it is possible to keep in contact with him too.

If my grandparents were to return to this earth, they would be utterly amazed to pick up a phone no larger than a pack of cigarettes and call anywhere they desired with no phone line connected.

The cell phone is only the beginning of how communications will change in the next fifty years.

Cell Phones 2

TO OUR AMAZEMENT, upon entering Mainland China, people in the cities were walking around with cell phones stuck to their ears. It seems as if the population has bypassed the conventional landlines because of the long waiting period for installation. With conventional phones, all types of lines ran around over the major and some minor cities. It troubled me to see the mess of lines above my head. The cell phone has answered this problem. Also, students and young adults enjoy having a phone that no other party can be connected to. I do not know this for sure, but is it possible that this is one way of getting around the censorship of the government?

In our present national government, the attorney general's office has deemed that it is not against our liberties to snoop into the phone calls we send and receive. This may be all right in a time of war, which the present administration says we are in, but most of our population does not see it that way.

Why have cell phones become so popular? Here are my thoughts: They are convenient to use, and they are always at your disposal. No one else can interrupt your conversation, and they appear to be relatively free from others listening in. They take the place of landlines and thus are supposed to save users money. With the right company, one can call any place in the United States or overseas.

What are the disadvantages? The biggest is that users need to be sure they don't go over the amount of time allowed under the program they purchased. If they do, the cost becomes very expensive. This is especially important with teenagers. They can talk, talk, talk, and talk some more without ever thinking about the cost. Talking is one thing teenagers do very well. They enjoy hearing the sound of their own voices. Teenagers also feel that with a cell phone they have complete privacy. They think that no one can listen to their conversations, especially if it is something they do not want the adults to hear about. What they do not understand is that others close by can hear their conversations. When teenagers become enthralled with their own talking, they forget everything else and thus lose track of someone else listening to them.

As I mentioned before, I think the major reason why cell phones sell is because of the convenience. You do not have to go to the location of a phone because you carry it on your person. The "Bluetooth" makes it especially convenient for a person driving down the highway to use the cell phone without having to take his or her eyes off the road or to hold the phone. This is a safety help. More and more the public authorities are concerned about the number of people listening and talking over their cell phones and thus not paying attention to their driving. Many accidents have been reported in the local press from such driving.

The air must be full of cell phone conversations all the time. It would be interesting to listen to the jumble that takes place as thousands of different messages go out into the air. The cell phone messages go to some relay tower to the next relay tower until they reach their destinations. I guess one could say that the cell phone is a small transmitter because it transmits different messages to different parts of the city, state, or world.

When did you purchase your first cell phone service? Ours began three or four years ago. Our first service experience was not happy at all, and we paid to get out of it. The next one we have had for over our contract time of two years, and we very recently purchased a service that is supposed to have the best coverage and the least-dropped calls in the United States. We hope the company is not lying to us. Thus far the service has been as presented.

Living in the western portion of the United States, we often have fewer privileges from companies; yet we also enjoy a better style of living—laid-back and not in a big hurry as is normal in the Midwest and on the East Coast.

Having in the last two weeks divested ourselves of a landline, we shall now see how the cell phone supplies our needs. One thing that is nice is that we are no longer pestered by salespeople at the meal hour or early in the morning or sometimes late at night. Now if the cell phone rings, we know it is a friend, a member of the church, or our immediate family. If only the Internet could or would figure out how to get rid of the "pop-ups," our lives would be much happier. Of course, I could shut off my Internet connection, but that would defeat the purpose for which I purchased the computer and Internet service.

In life, with the good comes the bad. One has to make decisions, and my decision to get rid of the landline was in an effort to eliminate the harassment that came as the baggage of the landline. Surely some individual is already thinking how he or she can grab my ear with the cell phone. I hope this person will not be able to do so.

The Internet

IT HAS ALWAYS amazed me how the Internet works. As I sit here at the keyboard of my computer and write these lines, others are writing lines on similar machines and sending the messages out into the air.

When did this all begin? Really, with the beginning of the twentieth century. This technology was always out there, yet only in this past century was it discovered. You see, the knowledge was there, but no one had been able to figure out how to harness it.

The push for the ability to send information out into space came about with the different governments attempting to get ahead and keep ahead of the others. Early on it was England and Germany in this struggle. Later on it was the United States and the Soviet Union battling, with missiles that sent the world into orbit, on how to get ahead and stay ahead of the other government. The United States government was ahead of Russia because one of the top German experts in this area decided that he preferred to be with the Americans rather than have his ability spent with the Russians.

The Internet was developed by our government to enable it to communicate swiftly and silently with the different branches. We wanted to be able to have immediate communication with our representatives all over the world. Working with coded messages, the different branches of our government around the world could communicate secretly without the other nations knowing what we were discussing or planning.

Other governments were soon using similar technology. Each government knew the others were communicating in this manner; thus, each of the governments had men and women working to break the codes of the other countries. The Internet and the computer became the backbone of such efforts. With these two instruments, each country could listen in on the secret thoughts of the others and attempt to break their codes to be ahead of those nations that were their enemies and sometimes those nations that were supposed to be friends.

This type of thing went on for years and still goes on. Some years ago the United States built a new embassy building in Moscow. Now, this in itself is nothing new. Each nation has its own buildings in other countries. What was different was that we learned that the Russian workmen who built the embassy installed sophisticated listening devices in the rooms. When our government moved in, at once the Russian government was able to hear our secret discussions. It soon became apparent what had taken place, and the building, which had cost us millions of dollars, was torn down.

Today the Internet and the computer, or some machine like it, are being used all over the world. The computer is the key to the Internet doing its work. Without the computer or similar machines, the Internet would be silent. It amazed me when I took my first computer class to learn that the messages going out over the Internet are made up of zeros and ones. How can combinations of these two numbers accomplish so much? I still do not understand it, but I use this process daily.

The Internet, much like the cell phone, has shrunk the world. We are now only a few clicks on a keyboard or a few numbers on a cell phone away from communicating with our friends or family thousands of miles away. All this change has come about because governments wanted to know what the other nations were doing to keep ahead of them or at least stay even. What would my grandfather think if he could come back and see the Internet?

Women Control Book Sales

RECENTLY I READ that women purchase 86 percent of the books sold in the United States. When I saw this, the question in my mind was, "Why?"

From what I've read, romance novels seem to be the main source of their purchases. Why does this happen? Are they unhappy in marriage? If they are not married, does such reading offer them the escape they need or want without having to pay the price of living with a partner?

Those of us who are married know that there are times when we wish we could escape from the obligations of marriage for a few days. If we truly gave our pledge for better or worse, this is not possible, and we use other means to escape. Reading romance novels may be one of the ways the female species live another life for an hour or two.

It is understandable that women desire to escape from the confines of household chores and the specifics of keeping children and a husband happy. Women think of having to satisfy a husband and children 365 days a year. Many women have three meals a day to be responsible for, clothes to wash, babies to diaper and feed, older children to care for, and a husband to keep satisfied sexually and romantically; a very difficult and taxing job for anyone. No wonder women escape into a romantic world!

Men, you ought to try preparing three meals a day for just one week. Do you think your wife would escape with a beer or glass of wine and watch a female program on the TV or curl up on the sofa with a romance novel while you prepared the meal? If you have a small baby, think of feeding him or her and keeping the baby happy with clean underclothes. If that is not enough, how would you like to satisfy the sexual and romantic desires of your wife when she comes home from a tough day in the office? Now you begin to understand the romance novel craze. All at once it is possible to leave the nagging boss or a cranky fellow worker as you bury your head in a book.

Yes, women do purchase 86 percent of the books in the USA. Many also watch the afternoon soaps. They are living each day in a different world through the eye gate, a book, or a TV soap.

I know of one lady who has her TV programmed to turn on the recorder to take down her favorite soap if she is not home to watch it in person.

Romance captures our sensual brain center and will not let go just like tobacco, which has been presented as romantic, does. I do not know if it is true, but a section I recently read stated that a student is captured by a cigarette if he or she takes one puff. If this is true, then the tobacco company has probably spent millions of dollars to learn how to fasten onto the physical and mental psyche of students before they realize they are addicted. Results from people who have been hooked on heroin indicate that cigarettes are more difficult to get off than hard drugs.

Psychologists have romanticized the use of certain drugs, especially tobacco. Women have been told in subtle ways that they look sexy and appealing when holding a cigarette. What we humans will do if we believe such an object makes us more appealing. How foolish we become to catch the attention of another human being. And often it is to no avail. Personally, beautiful women smelling of tobacco offend me. Their breath betrays the monkey on their backs. All the perfume in the world will not cover up the stench of tobacco in a person's body.

Escape in one form or another plays a large part in our addictions to romance, whether it is in the form of a book, a TV show, or a cigarette.

Why Do Men Feel Inferior to Women?

GOOD QUESTION. YES, why *do* men feel inferior to women? One reason is that women have more to do with the production of a child then men do. He plants the sperm that combines with the egg, and a fetus is produced. Men feel really detached from the whole process after the joy of planting the sperm. We feel as if we are bystanders, looking on as the process takes place. The woman is an active participant in the whole procedure. First, the female carries the baby; then, when the child is born, the woman uses all her body to bring forth the child into the space we know as the world; and after that, she feeds the child from her body.

Men also feel inferior to women because the female of the species is capable of taking over the process of rearing children from the word *go*. She can, if necessary, earn a living, run a household, and nourish the children until they reach adulthood. Perhaps men feel inferior because in some cultures the man has very little to do with the rearing of the children. The female is really in command of the total family operation; males are only standbys.

It's even worse for bees. In the bee culture, the male impregnates the queen bee and then dies. The workers and the queen take care of the new baby bees, providing their food and protection. Males are useless.

Moving further into the human culture, females directly communicate with the children by feeding, clothing, educating, and nurturing the children until they are able to care for themselves. Over the centuries men have been the hunters and protectors of their females, children, and elderly, but now it seems that females have taken over the role of family guardian.

In the past males protected their families and brought home the food; women prepared and cooked the food, washed the clothes, fed the babies, and generally supplied the foundation of their families. It is interesting to note that men died earlier than women, and males were remembered by how good they were at supplying the necessary food and staving off the enemy. Thus, men early on in civilization found themselves marginalized. The family, tribe, and country looked up to women, even though they allowed the men to flaunt themselves as the ones in the limelight.

I think we men have learned to put women down because we know that they hold a much higher place in the family or community. They just allow us to believe we are better. Only now are women really coming to the forefront in the United States' legislative branch of government.

In the secrets of our minds, I think we men have known all along that females could outdistance us if they decided to do so. Females may not have the physical strength of males, but they are wise in using the physical strength of the males to accomplish their needs. Long live the females of the species!

Cures

HAVE YOU EVER wondered what is behind the claims of certain products to cure all ills? Today, the claims on TV almost make it seem as if we have returned to the "snake oil days" of the last century, when certain salespeople claimed that their product would cure almost every disease known to mankind.

People have always been open to such claims. For example, Lydia Pinkham's bottled formula claimed it would help about every ailment a woman might have. I can remember seeing these bottles on the shelves of stores, not just drugstores, when I was a small boy. Interestingly, this medication generally contained a high percentage of alcohol, which is ironic since the women taking it were often members of the Women's Christian Temperance Union.

Other types of cures were claimed by the traveling evangelists who would lay hands on the sick, lame, or blind and claim that the person had been cured. Today we see these acts taking place on TV. The preacher will shout loudly and shove clients into the hands of the assistant. Are they cured? The clients will claim to be cured, but is there any follow-up?

Now, I am not saying that God will not and did not cure people of disease. He does and did. Jesus performed such cures while He ministered here on earth in the first century.

What is a cure? A cure seems to indicate that a person is set free from all the ills that have been associated with certain diseases. The person no longer has any of the effects known to have been part of the affliction.

Today, while acting as a volunteer chaplain in a hospital, I witnessed a poor soul wandering in and out of her room in her hospital gown, carrying all her clothes in a plastic bag, waiting to be taken home by friends. She was in a certain stage of dementia or, at the least, suffering from the symptoms associated with old age. I thought, *What cure is possible, outside of the intervention of God, for this poor soul?* She will continue to like this until her body wears out and she is buried. We do not know of any medical cure for such a disease. When a person's brain wears out, he or she becomes less of self—people begin to lose their identity. The person is no longer present. Another being has taken over residence in that "temple of clay."

Not all diseases, however, are without a cure. Actually, many marvelous cures have taken place in the human body thanks to modern medicine. God has given to man, through experimentation, remedies not known or even suspected in the last century. For example, pneumonia at its height was known as "the old man's friend." The old man died from its effects. My own great-grandfather died from this disease at a very early age, in his early forties, leaving a widow with five growing sons. Today he would be cured with the powerful medicines we have.

As I write these lines, I suffer from a severe curvature of the spine, inherited from both of my parents. It is painful all the time, and little seems to be able to cure it, partially because of my eighty-six years. My spine is so out of alignment and twisted that it cannot be remade by the surgeons, or they are afraid to attempt it. Two of the best in the city of Tucson have stated that they cannot help me.

On the other hand, my great-niece at an early age had rods placed along her spine, and today she stands tall and straight as a young lady of thirty years. This surgery was unknown in my early years, and my parents would not have had the money to have such surgery performed anyway.

How I wish they had a cure for my ailment. The pain is sometimes almost more than I can bear. Often the only relief I can find is to lie down on the floor, flat on my back, and stretch out. Most often this will help to relieve the pain. Oh, they do have medications to relieve the pain, but I am like a zombie after taking them. As they say of some drunks, "They were feeling no pain."

Even though in the medical world there are potential cures for some things and none for others, there is one sure cure here on this earth. We in the Christian faith know it as the cure for sin. This cure is forgiveness for our sins as we accept Jesus Christ as the ruler of our lives. We find the cure for sin in our belief in Him.

In many countries today, His followers are not known as Christians; rather they are known as "believers." No longer does identification as a Christian mean "born from above." It has many different meanings, all the way from saying, "I am a member of this denomination" to saying, "I pray every day" or "I believe in a divine power."

From the first century on, to proclaim you were a Christian meant that you accepted the teachings of Jesus Christ, believed in His death and resurrection as the way to salvation, and with the help of the Holy Spirit attempted to live as He taught.

This was the absolute cure from sin.

The Wonder of Our Age

EACH TIME I hit a computer key, the wonder of this age comes to mind. My grandfather and father would never have dreamed of such a piece of equipment. My generation has lived in a time of astonishing inventions. The telephone, telegraph, radio, TV, computer, and many other things have been invented in our lifetime.

The different pieces of electronic equipment our children and grandchildren use today boggles the mind. What is on the way for the future will be even more astonishing.

Starting with the "horseless carriage" at the turn of the century and now looking to power the automobile on hydrogen, strips the mind of its capacity to envision the possibilities in the future. Who knows what will be discovered. The recent gasoline shortage reminds us of the fact that fossil fuels will not go on forever. Also, the price can be expected to jump again in the near future. The US public has a short memory. The oil companies have made tremendous profits. I think the government should place a "windfall tax" on them.

Another wonder of our age is the airplane. To see a large airship full of passengers speed down the runway and slowly climb into the air is amazing. Mankind dreamed of this wonder for generations. As we saw the birds fly, catching the up drafts and downdrafts of air, we dreamed that one day we would do the same. Today we perform this wonder on a regular basis.

There are wonders in the medical profession. Wonders in surgery are daily coming to the attention of the public. Today, right this moment, surgeons are using robotic arms to enter bodies, perform the surgery, and retreat without a human hand ever entering the cavity. However, we have not been able to find a remedy for the common cold. We call it a "common cold," but when one has it, the cold is not too common.

In our time, eye surgery is very common. Different parts of the eye are operated upon and certain parts are replaced with plastic pieces. Individuals who have had this surgery remark that they can see better than when they used the original.

I saw only yesterday that surgeons are running a wire from the heart to the brain to help certain patients who are under much depression to overcome it.

Yet, with all of our progress, the only repair which can be made for sin is the conversion experience. Addicts of any type are still dependent for complete recovery upon the Lord Jesus Christ. The only sure solution for self-abuse is salvation through the power of God. We cannot lift ourselves by our own strength from the power of sin. It takes the power of God to perform this wonder, and it is a wonder to see the dramatic changes that occur in the lives of certain individuals. This wonder has been in progress since the day Jesus Christ placed His hand on the eyes of the blind man and told him he could see. The love Jesus showed to mankind while on this earth is a wonder that continues to change lives, momentarily and regularly.

Today we see that the power of God is in action all over the world. How? In people being saved from their sins. In the birth of a child, the healing of a cripple, or the restoring of sight to the blind. Often things like these last three are with the help of a medical person, but they are wonders from the hand of God.

Another wonder that takes place is the restoration of the relationship between a husband and wife or parents and their children. To see love come back into a home shattered by divorce is a wonder, just like seeing love come to spouses when either one or both of them have been unfaithful. These are wonders purchased by the Lord Jesus Christ in His death on the cross.

The hymn "O, what a wonder that Jesus loved me..." is true of each human being, for we have all come short of the glory of God (Rom. 3:23). He made us in His likeness and image, but through our free will, we have chosen to blacken that likeness.

The wonders of God and our generation boggle the mind!

Section Five

Christianity

Airline Hostess

SHE SAILED INTO the hospital lobby one day—a tall, erect African-American, who was a retired female airline hostess. Looking to enter a new profession, she was interested in the medical field and exploring what occupations might be open.

Over the next months, she came in often as a part of her moving into the field of a physician. This lady had a good academic background and had chosen to become an herbal specialist. Although we spoke often, our conversations never arrived at why she had chosen this field; they mostly centered on the manner in which people in the medical profession misuse themselves.

Then one day this fall we began to converse about religion and the Christian faith in particular. It turns out that we are both evangelical believers. Not shouting, hand-raising believers, but those who believe in the fundamentals of the faith—we know the meaning of being "born from above."

A sense of the presence of the Holy Spirit was evident between us. It is impossible to describe, but one feels and knows it is there, even as my wife and I felt it in services of worship while in Pakistan and China. Even though we could not speak or understand the language, there was that sense of the Holy Spirit's presence in the services of worship we took part in.

How did I sense His presence as we talked together in the lobby of the hospital? To be honest, I do not know exactly how to describe that sense. A strange awareness of the presence just took place as we communicated. Was it a sense of a sister and brother relationship, a closeness that went beyond the border of skin or nationality? Was it that we knew a person who is called Jesus Christ? How did this take place between total strangers?

This sense of the Holy Spirit's presence has always puzzled me when I have spent time going over it in the workings of my mind. Did the Holy Spirit arise from the unconscious portion of my intelligence? Questions and more questions; where are the answers? Is this how it will be in the afterlife when we are resurrected from the dead? Will we be united in the presence of God but have no sensual relationship between male and female? Is this what Jesus Christ meant when He told His disciples, "There is neither marriage nor given in marriage in the afterlife" (Matt. 22:30)?

As I sit here at my computer keyboard, my mind is traveling into the depths of its unconscious. Is that what is occurring at this very moment? What is it that takes place between this African-American lady and me? The relationship is not one of sexuality or just a sense of this meeting of souls; it is far beyond that. Yes, she is beautiful and stately, but there is a far different connection between this female and me. For one thing, I am many years her senior, and she probably has no feeling in this sense for me, or I for her. What is released between the two of us who claim Jesus Christ as our Savior and Lord?

Questions with no answers seem to be where I am going with this epistle. Why does this subject fascinate me? What is going on in my psyche? Puzzled, yes; answers, no. How can my mind wander into such depths, when it comes from no place in my conscious, but yet it must be present on some conscious level?

Airline Hostess

Strange, I cannot even recall her name. But there is a certain joy in the presence this total stranger, a strange, exotic joy. From where does it arise? Often we talk for some length of time until another person comes to the information desk asking for help. Does this lady desire the opportunity to share her thoughts with a kindred "believer"?

We had visited many times before, but it was only last time she visited that we came to the subject of both being "believers." Was this the work of the Holy Spirit? Sharing is witnessing, and witnessing takes place when the Holy Spirit opens the door. It doesn't work when we kick open the door. He has to know the exact time to turn the doorknob. It is then our duty to step through the open door and witness for Christ.

The next time I am on duty at the information desk, we shall have a different relationship because we both know Jesus Christ as our Savior. This is the tie my wife and I have found as we've met with different nationalities around the world. This is the tie we have with all believers.

What a privilege we have as members of the body of Christ.

Justice

WHEN YOU SAY the word *justice*, what comes into your mind? Do you see a criminal standing before a judge? If so, we hope he or she has a competent lawyer to represent him or her. Although if you are the person before the judge, sometimes even the best lawyer is not always able to assist you.

It is amazing to me to see all the things that the word *justice* means today; really, it all seems to depend on who is dealing with the justice system.

When I think of the word, judgment comes to my mind immediately. Judgment implies a decision being made either for or against an object or person. Is judgment one side of the coin of justice?

Antiques Roadshow, a PBS production, is built on the judgment of a supposed authority in a particular area of craftsmanship. In this show we see the surprise on the face of the owner of a particular item when he or she is told how much the item is worth, how old it may be, and whether it is authentic. Judgment is being made at that moment. The owner is either awed or downright surprised, and sometimes both.

Recently on TV, the shows with judges have been the rave of each network. On these shows people bring their grievances before the judge to have him or her decide what is proper in small claims court. One of the parties is going to be satisfied and the other dissatisfied. Both cannot be satisfied; it is not in the justice system.

Justice and judgment bring to my mind a picture of the last judgment, when all of mankind will be brought before God to give an account of how they used the life God granted them. As a child and in my teens, the preachers we had in the denomination in which I was reared pictured this day in vivid colors. These men of God believed you scared people into the kingdom of heaven. To this end, they made hell a reality. The hotter they could build the fire, the more converts hit the "sawdust trail."

Each year at a camp meeting, person after person would come to the altar to rehash their sins. These preachers believed in the Wesleyan doctrine of never knowing for sure if you were in or out of the kingdom of God. This is in contrast to the Calvinistic doctrine of eternal security. Once you are in the family, you are in the family, just as my sons and daughters are members of my family for life, sins and all.

A seventeenth-century preacher produced a sermon that had the listeners crying out for God's mercy when he preached. The sermon was called "Sinners in the Hands of an Angry God." This preacher made hell so real that his audience wanted nothing to do with it. Judgment was upon the members of the audience even as they listened.

Sometimes this is the concept I have as I listen to a televangelist. Many of them seem to believe they have to shout and prance about in order to get the attention of the audience. I believe God and people can hear them very well without the entire "theater act" being tossed in. Often I shut off the sound and watch these "actors" as they carry on. It crosses my mind, *What does God think of all this?*

Am I being judgmental or only asking a question? *Justice*—what does this word really mean in our society today? Has the meaning changed from the days when the Bible was placed in writing? Has our modern-day society twisted the meaning to satisfy its desires? Is there no black and white in our time?

Justice. What does it mean today?

Money

DOES THE USE or misuse of money cause strife between you and your spouse? According to the latest poll, the chief cause of divorce is misunderstandings about how the family funds should be used. Fortunate are the couples who before becoming one work through how they will use the money that comes into their hands.

My wife and I have always had only one purse, and from it we each spent as we decided together. In our family, because we are Christians and take the biblical admonition seriously, our tithe of 10 percent always came off the top of our income each month or quarter. We then decided how God was leading us to direct this percentage to His work. Both of us had tithed prior to our marriage, so this was something we decided we would do together as well. Because we made this conscious decision prior to our marriage, there was not a problem between us in relation to how the money that came into our hands was used.

Most of the time we have also been in agreement as to where the other money we received should be directed. In addition, we have been able to stay out of debt because we pay for each item when we purchase it. If we do not have the money to pay for the purchase at the time we want something, we do not buy it. This has remained true today with our debit card; we know what we pay for at the moment we enter into the contract to acquire it. We do not have monthly payments to make.

Many in this nation are in debt and extended beyond their limits because they do not pay for each item as they buy it. Even the homes being sold today are paid for on a monthly basis. And some people are not even paying on the principal, only the interest; not one cent is being applied to the principal. In reality, the home never belongs to the purchaser, but it resides in the hands of the lending institution.

With these types of financial situations, if one of the family members is laid off or becomes seriously ill and the money of one paycheck does not come in, the family is quickly in financial trouble. No wonder we have so many people with serious mental health problems in our nation! It is estimated that 20 percent of our population is depressed at any one time with some seriously depressed. If the statistics are correct, 5 to 10 percent of the population is on medication for depression.

The sad thing is that young people copy the way in which their parents have unwisely spent their money. The children of these families follow the same example. The bank card companies are also to blame for this financial situation. They flood these teens with credit cards, thus continuing the financial problems prior to their coming to adulthood.

I have watched this situation in my own immediate family. My grandchildren had huge debts when they were hardly into the age of adulthood. One grandson is even now paying off debts he acquired while in college—both college loans and other personal debts.

It is not just the individuals of our nation who are in debt; our nation as a whole is in deep financial trouble because we have overextended our use of the tax dollars that come into the federal, state, and county treasuries. Our Congress spends money as if there is no end of it. The members of Congress do not have the backbone to tell their voters, "This is all the money we have to use, and we will not borrow more." Do they do this? No! They feel they must give in to every whim of their people to win their seat in the Congress. Our national debt goes higher and higher because these members will not say no.

Yet even as a family can go into debt only so far, so also the Congress is going to reach the end of its borrowing limits. Today China, Japan, and England own us. Why? Because they have purchased our bonds in huge numbers, so much so that we are now in debt over our government limits. If they decide not to buy our bonds anymore, we shall be in severe financial trouble. And just as in a family, the national finances can operate only a certain length of time in the red before the world comes crashing down around our financial heads.

My memory is very good. I lived into and through the Great Depression that began in 1929. We are following the same pattern now that caused our money to be worthless then. Germany went through this after World War I. This was the reason Hitler was able to take over. A desperate people will resort to desperate measures. And when a family is dependent upon a weekly paycheck to exist and the paycheck does not arrive, then families may begin to fall apart.

Money! The Bible tells us that the love of money is the root of all evil (1 Tim. 6:10). It is not the money that is the problem; it is the wrong perspective or misuse of it. Sadly, many Christian people have become involved in the web of the financial spider now crippling our nation. Fortunate is the couple who place God *first* in the use of the funds He allocates to them. The Scriptures tell us, "But seek ye first the kingdom of God, and his righteousness; and all these things shall be added unto you" (Matt. 6:33 KJV).

Money. Are you a good steward?

Will We Be Married in Heaven?

MANY PEOPLE ARE asking this question today because of the emphasis the Mormons or the Church of Jesus Christ of Latter-day Saints place on celestial marriage. They say that you will have the same wife in heaven that you have on this earth. Jesus Christ, in response to this question, said two thousand years ago, "You are neither married nor given in marriage" (Matt. 22:30).

Polygamy fits into the theology of the Latter-day Saints (LDS) because they believe God was once a man as you and I and had a goddess wife. The two of them had sexual relations and produced many children, who came to earth through men and women having sexual relations on this earth. Polygamy supplied the many wives needed to bring down these celestial children and thus fulfilled the belief of the LDS church that all men and women, if they live rightly, can become gods and goddesses.

Mormon theology states, "As god once was, so we can become." Their belief is that God, as we know Him, was once a human being and progressed in His spiritual life until He became a god. They believe that men and women can progress in godliness until we die, and then we will have a planet we can rule as the gods or goddesses of the universe.

Some Mormons in remote areas of the United States, especially in the Southwest, are practicing polygamy in our time. Currently, a splinter branch of the LDS church is under arrest for sponsoring the doctrine of polygamy. An LDS elder arranged it so that a fourteen-year-old female was married to a man in his forties. For years it has been known that splinter groups of the LDS faith have lived in this situation. But because they are in remote areas of the nation, nothing has been done about these types of relationships.

If you buy into this LDS concept, then you would have no trouble, whether as a male or female, being a part of polygamy. Polygamy was practiced in the early history of nations, partially because the males had been killed off in wars and because even in the normal span women outnumbered men. If one man could support many wives, then the females would not be left to starve to death or lack offspring. This was a disaster in the early religious life. Children were procreated because they were the social security of the day and hour.

In contrast, China is in trouble today because they allowed only one child in a family in an attempt to control their population growth. If the one child turned out to be a female, she was aborted or killed upon birth. Now the Chinese have too many males and not enough females to meet the needs of those in the male population who desire to marry. To meet the need for females, efforts are being made to bring in females from other nations. Strange as it seems, you can't fool "mother nature."

To further complicate this marriage picture, as the Chinese population moves from the rural areas to the cities, many females are finding employment and have decided to stay single. Because of the abuse females have taken in the male-dominated culture, many females who know they can survive alone are saying, "I don't want to be married. Singleness is good enough for me. Why should I put up with emotional and physical abuse?"

It is easy to understand their reluctance to enter into a marriage contract. Females have been the pawns of males for centuries in the Chinese culture. No longer is this necessary when the women can supply their own physical needs; they need not be dominated by an uncaring male companion.

Many people who have heard the Mormon theology or of situations like the one in China will be happy to hear the response of Christ to the question by the religious leaders of His day. These people are saying, "I do not want to be married here on earth to the person I'm with now. Why would I want to be married to that individual in the afterlife?"

One of my Christian friends gave the best response I have heard in a long time to this question about marriage in heaven when she said, "I will know the person in heaven, but I will not have the same emotional attachment that I had here on earth."

According to Scripture, if a female is not married here on earth, then she does not need to worry about being married in the afterlife. God made marriage between a man and woman for two reasons: 1) to furnish a helpmate for the males, 2) to continue populating the earth. In heaven this is not needed. We shall have many, many friends, and there will be no need to have sexual relations to populate heaven.

Will you be married in heaven? Jesus Christ, the only Son of God, stated point blank: no. "At the resurrection people will neither marry nor be given in marriage; they will be like the angels in heaven" (Matt. 22:30).

O Little Town of Bethlehem

FOR ME AS a child, Christmas was a seminal event of the year. We all sang Christmas carols and enjoyed every minute of it. Christmas has now become very commercial, but happily there are still millions of us who enjoy the reason for the season. Celebrating the birth of Jesus Christ brings hope to thousands, maybe even millions of children and to those who want to remember their childhood.

Our society has so romanticized the season that it becomes difficult to remember the reason we celebrate it. It is sad when merchants count on the Christmas season to produce 40 percent of their income for the financial year. Because of the excessive spending that takes place at this season, individuals and families suffer the remainder of the next year. Husbands and wives have real knock-down, drag-out affairs because of their overspending at Christmastime. Credit cards are maxed out; payments become a burden on the family because of the overextension in their financial situation. "Glory to God in the Highest" is not the song that is sung when the credit card payments become due. Financial struggles take place, and sometimes merchandise has to be returned because our financial eyes are larger than our financial stomachs.

Salt and Pepper

Our economy is based on spending and buying, not on keeping and using over and over again. I am sorry to say that I can remember when all this began to take place. It was when the government and companies urged people to take on debt. If the national government could stay in debt all the time, why not urge the people to do the same?

Today our nation finds itself so in debt to China, Japan, and England that we must keep running at breakneck speed just to pay the interest on the bonds the US government has sold to these nations.

"O little town of Bethlehem, how still we see thee lie!" Now terrible fighting is taking place because of what happened in that backwater town. The Christian faith and, to a larger extent, the business world of the United States is face-to-face with an enemy birthed by the Islamic world. The Muslims are out to bring the world as we know it under their complete control. They almost did it in the sixteenth century. Today they are on the march again, financed by the oil needs of the Western world.

The "Little Town of Bethlehem" is seen as a source of revenue for the Islamic world in Palestine. Until the struggle began between Jews and the Palestinians of the radical Islamic world, merchants in this little town made a decent living from the flood of evangelical Christians wanting to travel the roads Jesus Christ did. Now Muslims populate this little, dirt street town. Evangelical Christians still want to see the holy places written about in the Bible, and other sacred and secular people desire to do the same. Thus, we now feed the Muslims' financial stomachs.

Unless the Muslim society changes, the streets of Bethlehem will not ring with the happy voices of Christians marching to their favorite historical sites.

Mankind longs for the peace written about in the Bible, but as long as mankind uses his free will to cause other countries trouble, peace will not arrive.

How we long for the Prince of Peace to return as He promised.

The Supernatural

AS I WAS making my rounds in the hospital as the volunteer chaplain, I met a blind man and his sister. I came into the room and introduced myself as the Protestant chaplain and noticed that this man was fingering a toy red eighteen-wheeler.

The sister began to converse with me, all the time keeping a hand or, I should say, he was keeping a hand on his sister's arm. As we spoke, the sister informed me that her brother could feel colors. She told me of how he touched his brother-in-law's new truck and said, "You have a white truck." This lady and her husband had purposely not told the brother the color to see how he would respond.

Lying before him on a table was a green-covered, loose-leaf notebook. He had identified it as green. A person who was acquainted with the blind told the sister that colors give off certain vibes, and this was what her brother could read about colors. The sister said he never missed.

I wondered, *What supernatural powers does this man possess?* His speech was limited, and the sister told me that it took all her strength to take care of her brother. Because she was so worn out from the 24/7 care required and was battling both cancer and lupus that were reappearing, he had been placed in a care facility. He was in the hospital only because three red lines began running up his right arm, which indicated infection. This had been cleared up in the hospital, and he would soon be going back to the care facility.

She continued to tell me about her brother. She said that he had been placed in the School for the Blind. There he had quickly learned to use the cane that we see the blind using all the time. His sense of the supernatural had made it possible for him to learn in a few short days the correct use of his white cane, while others took much longer.

As I stood there listening to his sister, the blind brother would run his fingers up and down her arm. This seemed to give him a sense of safety. His sister informed me that she had taken care of him for many years until he became too much for her with the limitations lupus and cancer had placed on her. Perhaps a certain bond had taken place between the brother and sister that gave them a type of mutuality.

Often you see some type of connection occur between husband and wife, one in which no words are spoken; yet they understand what the other person means. A lifted eyebrow, a tilt of the head, the set of the mouth, or the placing of the arms all indicate unspoken messages.

Meeting this man and his sister made me think. What senses do the visually impaired have that we do not seem to have? Or is it that we do not need to cultivate that capacity? Perhaps all of us have this capacity, but because we are visual, we do not have to depend upon it. Could it be that we all have this supernatural capacity but seldom use it? This would make a good doctoral study for a student in psychology. How would such a study be set up, and what results would the study look to prove or disprove?

Those who have studied animals tell us that they have certain sounds that they utter and that members of the same species understand. God has given to all His animal creation the capacity to communicate, each of the species in different ways. Perhaps this is what takes place with the human and the supernatural. Who knows for sure?

God Works in Mysterious Ways

THE POWER OF prayer is echoed in the Scriptures when James states, "The prayer of a righteous man is powerful and effective" (James 5:16). This past week this writer has seen this come true. Our sixty-one-year-old daughter was stricken with TIA, a short-term memory loss. The medical people say that this takes place when a small blood clot hits the brain in a certain place. This causes the brain to malfunction and may cause serious damage. Fortunately, this did not occur with our daughter. She is now, from all signs, completely recovered.

The process of healing was taking place even as the prayers were being offered and before the neurologist saw our daughter. God was answering the flood of prayers that were going up to Him from many different sources. From 10:30 in the morning until 4:00 in the afternoon, our daughter did not know what took place. Then very slowly her short-term memory began to return. By evening, she had almost completely recovered from her loss. Only a small portion of the loss remained.

Often we do not see the action of God because sometimes answers to prayers are not as dramatic as this. But it thrills us Christians when we see the results of our prayers take effect so rapidly. However, we need to remember that God is still working when we do not see His actions as quickly. God doesn't *not* answer prayers. He always answers, perhaps just not in the way we expect or the way we want Him to. His plan of answering and ours may be on very different timetables. In our daughter's case, He knew that if she was to fully recover, His actions needed to be immediate; thus He acted.

A very positive thing came out of this incident. My daughter's husband and youngest son saw the response God made to the prayers. They do not claim to be deep believers in Jesus Christ, even though both of them know the Way. Actually, each of the people affected by the TIA of our daughter knew the truth of salvation through Jesus Christ, but some are not willing to let Him become the Master of their lives. From the very early years of their lives, they have heard the Word preached and taught in Sunday school classes, yet they have not allowed Him to be completely in control. This action on the part of our daughter's youngest son has cost him dearly, but he still continues to stay outside the fold of God.

In contrast, the eldest son, a truck driver, told his mother that he had made an agreement with God. Apparently he is sticking with his agreement. He never told his mother what it was, but it has changed his life. He has become very active in the United Methodist Church close to where he lives and has found a lady to be his wife. Now, I know going to church does not indicate you are a Christian, but his actions since that date seem to indicate this to be true.

Though we cannot see it, often good comes out of what we humans see as evil. Let us hope this is the case in the TIA of our only daughter. Further, it is our hope that many people will be won to Christ because of this incident and the manner in which the Creator of men and women acted at once.

Thoughts on Dying

TWELVE COAL MINERS died. Twelve families are left without husbands, fathers, grandfathers, and lovers. The news only reports the facts. How does the news report the horror and agony of the miners and their families?

Seeing these emotions played out on TV reminded me of the fact that I have outlived the normal seventy-two years for United States males. Our age group is the fastest growing section of the population. No longer must the merchants place all their attention on the youth of our nation.

Having already come very close to death in October of 2004 while on a visit to China, it no longer holds horror for me. Preferably, it would be my desire to go to be with the Lord in my sleep, but that exercise will be in His power. No one desires to die in a great deal of pain, including me.

This Christmastime, in an effort to remind our children that we are not going to live forever, we gave each of them a copy of our living will. We had previously shown them where our wills are to be found, in the lockbox in the walk-in closet off the master bedroom. We also have a paper from the memorial society we belong to that indicates the steps our children should take in the event of our death. As members of this memorial society, for $545 we can have our bodies carried to the mortuary and cremated. Our children do not desire to believe that we will not live forever, but this is a fact. Thus, we needed to acquaint them with the facts of death as they relate to their parents. I do not want to see the small bit of money I have in the bank help a mortician purchase a new Rolls-Royce.

My experiences with death have been through my parents going to be with the Lord. The evening I walked into the funeral home in a small town in Michigan, walked up to the casket, and looked into the face of the body of my father is still fresh in my mind. In my pastoral experience, I had been called upon to preside at the memorial services for members of the congregations where I had served. However, these experiences had not prepared me for the death of my own flesh and blood. The stark reality that I would never see this person again on this earth hit me like a sledgehammer. This was the final act in the play related to my father's eighty years on this earth. Only a shell was in the casket; Dad was not present. He was now in the presence of God.

Ten years later, I stood and looked at the grave marker in this same small Michigan town, where my father was buried. My mother had been laid to rest beside the body of Dad. I talked with her and wept as I stood looking at the earth where the woman who bore me, loved me, and defended me was placed. It had been impossible for me to return to that small Michigan town for her memorial service because of a terrible snowstorm, which occurred in December of 1990.

Mom had recently reached her eighty-ninth year. She had suffered stroke after stroke after stroke, and she was no longer the person who loved me. She was like an animal in the last years of her life. All sense of her womanhood had vanished. But the glory of it all was that Mom knew the Lord Jesus Christ as her Savior. There was never any doubt about that. I can still hear her singing the gospel songs she had leaned on as a child as she worked in her home. These hymns were the guiding spirit in her life and kept her sane when insanity was part of the household.

She was thoroughly committed to a belief in Jesus Christ as He was presented in the King James Version of the Bible.

The finality of her death reminded me again of the truths I had been taught as a child and into manhood. I was taught that Jesus Christ went to prepare a place for those who trusted His teachings and believed what He had taught His disciples while on this earth.

Jesus said, "I go to prepare a place for you, that where I am, you may be also." He also stated, "In my Father's house are many rooms." This indicated the huge size of the place He had prepared for those who believe in Him. He told the thief on the cross on the day He was crucified, "Today you will be with me in Paradise." We need to hear these Scriptures because we are in a time when death is all around us, and many people in the world's population are dying horrible deaths.

Someone stated, "Two things are for certain, death and taxes." I do not argue with this at all. My only hope is that the Lord will take me from this house into His house while I sleep.

Gift Giving

AS I GATHERED with the rest of the people purchasing gifts, these thoughts occurred to me: *What is the meaning of this? How have the merchants taken over a sacred time for a secular business opportunity? As Christians, how and why have we allowed them to do this? Are we as guilty as they in allowing the secular world to take over a sacred time? Have we joined in as we've rushed to purchase gifts?*

A few years ago I watched our grandchildren tear off the packaging of the gifts they had received at Christmastime and then toss the gifts aside as they scrambled to pick up another. They had so many gifts that they did not know what to do with all of them. Yes, we adults were responsible for their frenzy. Stacking all the gifts under the Christmas tree made it impossible for the child to understand what was taking place.

My understanding is that merchants expect to receive almost one-half of their income from business in the Christmas season. What does this say about our value system? Families will overextend their credit line and struggle to meet the minimum payments on their credit cards for the next year. Why do we allow this frenzy of buying to exhaust us?

My wife and I have decided to limit our buying to that product that will be of value for the total year, instead of only one day. We give publications that will arrive each month, reminding the receiver of the value we place on him or her as family and friends. As a matter of fact, historians tell us that the date we observe for the time Christ came to this earth is not the date He arrived. We may be a number of years off in our calculations.

We adults enjoy saying; "Christmas is for children; that is why we take part." Are we all children, even in our adult skin? Gift giving came about because of the improbable gift that God gave to humankind in the person of Jesus Christ. Folks in the Christian faith know this, but what of the other human beings living on earth? Do they understand the reason for the season? Perhaps our abundance of income and things has blinded us to the reason for the season.

God, in His self-emptying love, sent Jesus Christ to this earth. This gift allowed humankind to see how deeply God loves each of us. When the Godhead decided to send a part of itself to live on this earth in the form of a man, this was a limitation we humans could not grasp. Coming as a baby, as each of us does, meant Christ took on the form of a human; worked at hard manual labor, spent three years walking over the roads and paths of Palestine, teaching, healing, and preaching; and was killed by the religious authorities of the day because they could not or would not understand this self-emptying love.

Secularism did not start recently; it has always been at work in this sacred season. Today we have enlarged it, but the same greed is still there that started two thousand years ago.

Question: Why do you give gifts at this time of the year? Is it a Christian privilege or part of the secular craze?

Helping Others

IN OUR DEVOTIONS this morning, the central thought was helping the needy. This caused me to remember a recent time when a woman came up to me in the Wal-Mart parking lot, asking for money for food. I turned her down. A few moments later a thought struck me like a sledgehammer: *You are to help the needy. It is the money of the Lord, and He emphasized our responsibility as His followers to help those in need.*

In situations like these, my reaction has always been, "How do I know how they will use the money?" But this is not my responsibility. Of course, if the person is drunk or on drugs, then this concept would not apply; but otherwise, how they use the Lord's money is their problem. He has given me more than enough, and now it is my turn to be a good steward of the funds He has bestowed upon my spouse and me. What I shall do from now on is take those who are asking for money and feed them. If they refuse, then I shall know the money they wanted was not for food but for some other purpose.

Some people make a very decent living "panhandling." Other folks are really in hard times and need any relief their fellowmen can give them. The sad thing is that most families are only two paychecks away from being out on the street. It is not only single people; today it is also families and often women with children whose husbands have left them to fend for themselves.

Housing in our city is costly; thus, those folk who come here in the wintertime find it impossible to have any type of housing except through the charity organizations. Apart from asking for help, these folks can also go the Salvation Army, the gospel rescue mission, or Catholic charities and receive help. Some of these charities aid people and tell them they must make an effort to help themselves too. For example, the Salvation Army (SA) demands that people get out on the street each day and look for work.

The SA people must be servants of the Lord to be able to work with problems day after day without "burning out." In my years of counseling it often became difficult for me to "keep my cool" when dealing with those who pictured themselves as helpless.

The Lord Jesus Christ had compassion on the poor, but even He in His human moments had to go up to the mountains for time away from the crowds to talk to His Father in heaven. Those of us who work in the helping world need to remember the example of the Lord, giving ourselves time to refresh; we should not "burn the candle at both ends."

A major problem in the ministry today is burnout, partially because we try to depend upon ourselves all the time and forget the power that will come to us through the channel of prayer. Talking to the Lord about how to proceed is number one in the refreshment schedule of those working in the ministering and helping professions. Listening to Him through the power of the Holy Spirit will give the minister or helping person the needed wisdom in each situation.

Often when counseling I found myself sharing from the depths of my soul thoughts that came from the Holy Spirit, for it was not in my understanding of the situation. Afterward I would marvel on how the Lord had stepped in and directed the counseling period. That moment when the counselor understands how God has acted is a real joy; the counselor is thrilled to be used by God to help his fellow human beings.

Long before the counseling profession, as such, came into being, the Scriptures record how certain prophets helped different people. If these situations are recorded in the Bible, there must have been many other times when God's helpers were active in helping their fellowmen.

A couple of years ago, as my spouse and I were about to enter Furr's Cafeteria, a man came up to me, asking for money for food. My response was "I'll take you inside and pay for a meal." He could not refuse because I had taken him at his word. The manager of the cafeteria asked if the man was bothering me. My reply was no, but the man who asked for help ate his meal quickly and was out of sight as soon as possible.

When I was a pastor, people came to the church office, asking for help. Because our congregation gave money to the Salvation Army, they were referred to them for assistance. Whether they went there we never knew, but at least we had made the attempt to help. Of course, this response was a convenient way to get rid of people.

The local congregation where we now worship has a community cupboard that the pastor or church secretary takes food from to help needy people who come to the door of the church. In times past, the church has helped families by paying their rent. These funds have come from the deacon's fund. We give to this fund often. Again, this is being a good steward of the money God has given us. The money we use is not ours; we are allowed to use it under the direction of the Holy Spirit—we need to listen to Him.

Jesus said, "The poor you have with you always." This is a truth we cannot escape. In our nation alone, a wealthy nation, at this moment 46.6 million people do not have any health insurance. These people are forced to go to hospital emergency rooms, which in turn cause the medical expenses to rise.

Helping the needy is how hospitals, mental institutions, and charity organization came into being through the direction of the Lord. He never seems to give up on helping His children, and we are all His children.

The Power of Prayer

HAVE YOU EVER felt as if your prayers went no farther than the ceiling? Often it seems as if mine hardly rise above the chair I am sitting in or the bed I am lying on. (I have assumed all positions suggested by those who are known for getting through to God.)

Prayer is talking to God as you would talk to your close friend, right? Do you ever feel your close friend must be off on a holiday? When I am in the "desert stage" of my prayer life, I use prayers from our *Book of Common Worship*. Other times I find hymns, which are prayers, and they express what I want to convey to God. Because God is my only true friend, He can talk to me through various means, whether in written prayers by another Christian, a particular hymn, a portion of Scripture, the music of a bird as it chirps, the morning sunrise, or the glorious sunsets we enjoy in Arizona.

Sometimes my prayers seem to be very personal, coming from the very depths of my soul. Other times it appears as if I am just mumbling words. Recently it has been my pattern to open my mouth and see what the Holy Spirit causes me to utter. At other times my expression to God is "You know more about me than I do. Please work on that which needs to be opened to me." It is my feeling that He sees into every corner and crevice of my subconscious; thus, He knows me better than I know myself.

Because I was reared in a tradition where the Lord's Prayer was part of every worship service and the morning devotions we had in my parental home, it is still a part of my daily prayers. Lately, I have been attempting to sense or feel, whatever you may want to name it, the depth of meaning when I say, "Our Father, who art in heaven…" Does this mean He is a long way away, or is it only me? When I speak the words "Our Father…" my mind transitions to the picture I have of Jesus Christ as presented in the New Testament. The Old Testament picture of God shows more of a God who is fierce and unkind, but Jesus stated, "Anyone who has seen me has seen the Father" (John 14:9). The God seen here is One who is loving, kind, forgiving, not given to hatred or harshness, and always on my side, if I allow Him to be.

It is an absolute necessity for me to go to the vision I have of Jesus in seeing God. The God I see in Jesus Christ is not weak, simpleminded, or a sissy. He is strong, not a pushover, has complete understanding of where I am coming from, does not look with favor on my sins, and yet is very willing to forgive me when I acknowledge them.

What is your perspective on God and prayer? Do you pray? It appears from polls that most citizens of the USA pray every day and that we who pray feel some success in our prayers. How about you? Is your prayer life dead in its tracks?

Why I Am a Christian

WHY I AM a believer (Christian) is partially because I was born into a Bible-believing family. Now I am a believer, as the Chinese brothers say, because it is the way of life I choose. I came to believe in the death and resurrection of Jesus Christ as the Son of God. The Christian life is a life of satisfaction, happiness, and the knowledge that when I leave this earth I shall live in the presence of God for all time, for eternity—that is, forever and ever.

What are the benefits of being a "believer"? First and foremost, we can find forgiveness through praying to God and asking for forgiveness for our sins. Our forgiveness is complete because of what Jesus Christ did on the cross; He paid the price for our sins so that we can be forgiven. It all sounds very simple, and it is, except we have to be willing to say that we need Christ to forgive us. Humility is the key here. But the free will that God gave humans when He created us stands in the way of our being humble enough to ask for forgiveness. The pleasure of sin—and it has its pleasures—causes us to turn from God and follow the way of the Evil One. The Evil One knows our weakness and slips in to turn our minds to evil. When the Holy Spirit causes us to see that we have sinned, then comes the moment of being humble enough to ask God to forgive us.

Even though we know God only wants the best for us, we often listen to Satan and follow his path. His path leads to destruction. He blinds our eyes so we do not see the canyon we are about to fall into. After we have followed the destructive path for so long, we lose sight of the good God has for us. Sin then becomes a way of life, and unless our minds are corrected, we follow this to our destruction and hell.

The problem with mankind is that we believe we have to do something to gain God's forgiveness, and we do; we have to be willing to humble ourselves and ask for it. There is no amount of good works that will purchase this forgiveness. We cannot work our way into eternal life with God and His followers. We have to accept His *free* gift. We cannot see this free gift. We are blinded by our sinful ways. We enjoy sinning. Mankind enjoys going against God, that is, until we give ourselves freely to Him.

When we actually do become servants of God, we do so freely, not because He forces us or chains us to Himself. We make the choice by our own free will. The free will He gave us at the time of our creation, and that we used against Him, we now use to turn our lives over to Him.

As believers, we find joy and satisfaction in living our lives for God. We have the presence of the Holy Spirit living in us. How do I know this? Jesus Christ told His disciples that He would send the Comforter, even the Holy Spirit, to live in each one of them (John 14:16). This applies to us too. When we allow God through Christ Jesus to make His home in our souls, the Holy Spirit comes to live in each believer. We are no longer walking down the path of life alone. The Holy Spirit is present to help us through the rough and tumble of living on this earth.

Not only do we have the reward of the guidance of the Holy Spirit on this earth, but we also have the sure knowledge of an eternal home with God in the afterlife. How do we pay for this? There is no possible way. Fortunately, Jesus already paid the price on our behalf.

Why I Am a Christian

Being a Christian is a life full of satisfaction in which we find forgiveness from sins when we confess them, have the presence and guidance of the Holy Spirit, and get to live forever in the presence of all that is good when we die.

All that I have written does not say that we shall not have troubles, sorrows, and heartaches on this earth, but we do not go it alone. Jesus Christ said, "Lo, I am with you always, even unto the end of the world" (Matt. 28:20 KJV). Being a believer ensures the presence of Christ always. We do not go it alone.

This is why I'm a Christian.

Angels

DO YOU BELIEVE in angels?

Many people believe in angels and other "ethereal" beings. Do you ever wonder why humankind desires to know about bodies which are outside our comprehension? Some religious groups pray to saints, believing that this is a more immediate way to gain the attention of God. But in Scripture we are taught that only going through Jesus Christ do we have direct access to God (1 Tim. 2:5). We do not need any other being to gain His attention.

The Bible speaks of angels both in the Old and New Testaments. Angels come in what appears to be human form. This is seen in the Old Testament when the angels came to Abraham after Sarah and he had prayed for a man-child. (God had promised Abraham he would have descendants as many as the sands of the sea or the stars of the heavens [Gen. 15:4].)

Genesis 18 says that the angels came as travelers on the pathway to the place where Abraham had his tent pitched, and he hurried out to meet them. This was the custom of hospitality in that region of the world. In some places a person can stay in a home for a period of three days with no questions asked, but then that person must move on, thanking the host for his graciousness. So Abraham was being a typical host to the angels in the form of men. These men, however, told Abraham that by the same time next year, Sarah and he would have a man-child born of their intercourse.

Now Sarah, hiding behind the tent flap, laughed at this ridiculous statement. One of the angels confronted Sarah, asking her, "Why did you laugh when I told your husband you would have a son, born from the two of you at this time next year?"

Of course Sarah, now afraid, said, "I did not laugh."

The angel replied, "I heard you laugh." Thus, we see that the angels can speak and are recognized as human beings, even though they really are spokesmen from God.

In the New Testament (Acts 12), when Peter was chained in the inner cell, an angel loosed him and spoke to him, and they hurried out the prison door. As a matter of fact, the angel took Peter out into the city, where Peter could find his way to the house where followers of Jesus were praying for his release, and then the angel disappeared.

When Peter appeared at the door of the home where the prayer meeting was taking place, the maid that came to the door in response to Peter's knock recognized his voice and ran to tell those inside that Peter was at the gate. The group thought she was seeing an angel. It took some convincing to get the group to allow Peter to come in, but they finally opened the gate and "were astonished." Even though the group had been praying for his release, it seems they did not believe their prayers had been answered.

When Jesus was a baby, the Holy Spirit came to Anna and Simeon in the temple and told them that the baby in the arms of Mary was the longed-for Messiah. Simeon believed and praised God, stating, "I have seen the Messiah, and now I can die in peace." Anna, the old prophetess, also declared she had seen the Messiah and that this baby was the longed-for Redeemer foretold by the prophets of old (see Luke 2).

The miraculous birth of Jesus Christ took place after an angel came to Mary, informing her of the process that would take place as the Holy Spirit caused her to be pregnant with the Son of God. Also, an angel told Joseph, who was betrothed to Mary, that Mary was clean and that he should not reject her because the child she was carrying was from God.

Angels are still appearing and working today. *Guideposts* has a sister publication called *Angels*. This magazine records incidents of angels working in our day and time to bring about miraculous acts in human beings. These are often stories of angelic bodies in human form.

Angels are for real. Has one ever visited you or your friends?

The Lord Returns

OUR WESTERN SKIES paint glorious pictures each day. Yesterday morning when we went walking, the sun was shining through the clouds. It was a brilliant display of God at work in His universe. No artist could have painted such a magnificent view. As I looked at the glory of the sky, I remembered the words of the Lord. Speaking to His disciples as He ascended into the heavens He said, "As you have seen me go, I shall come again in like manner."

I believe that someday Jesus will return in the manner in which He said He would. It makes me want to cry and shout when I visualize this return. How our world needs the return of the Lord. I am sure other generations have felt the same way, but our times seem to cry out even more for His immediate return.

My grandfather, who died eighty-five years ago, believed he would never die. He believed the Lord would return before he went to be with God. As we all can see, this has not taken place; the Lord has not come back yet.

As we look at history and our world today, we can see and understand the desperate need humanity has had over the generations since the Lord made that statement as He returned to be with the Father. Thinking people know that the human race is filled with sin; every way we turn we find is vital evidence of this. We cannot bring about peace; we are all too tied up in the power of evil.

Why God allows Satan to rule the world, I cannot understand. All Satan does is fill individual and national lives with tragedy. In our times, good seems to be taking a beating. Of course, this was also true in previous generations. This is the perception I have from reading history, both secular and sacred—the Khan hordes swept across Asia, and the Vikings terrorized the seacoast of Europe and maybe even were in the New World before Columbus arrived. It seems that each generation has Satan in a human form striking terror into the lives of common folks.

Thinking about all this, it is no wonder that I could visualize the sudden return of the Lord as I looked into the sky with all its brilliance this morning! In my lifetime, we have had one despot after another terrorizing the world with their satanic acts. People outside the Christian faith desire a change for the better as much as we within the body of Christ do, but they do not have any hope, except for in the vain efforts of a few men and women who are working to change our society with human means.

The United Nations was established with the concept in mind of doing for society what one nation could not or would not attempt. It seems to be a group of men and women who are powerless, except to pass resolutions. When it comes to taking action to help the needs of the common man, they only talk; there is no direction in this group.

The Roman Catholic Church with its billion plus members seems to be powerless to change society, even though it is the largest body of "believers." On the other side of the coin, Islam, with its one billion adherents is attempting to change society by force, using all the powers of destruction to bring about a world that fits their picture of what this world should be.

Both the church and the Muslims use the name of God and attempt to deal with evil in the world on a power basis. As long as this is their view of how to change society, humankind will journey in a swamp.

Both groups say they invoke the power of God, but in reality this is not so. They both act in a manner only common to human thinking.

An old hymn I remember states, "Sunrise tomorrow, sunrise tomorrow, when in His beauty I see the great King." All through the Bible, both the Old and New Testaments proclaim that this day shall come when evil is destroyed. When I see the sun shining through the white clouds in our blue western sky, His return seems very positive to me. How about you? When you see such a picture, does your mind conjure up the end time?

Short-Timer

DO YOU KNOW what a "short-timer" is? In the armed forces, a service person who has a limited time in his enlistment is known as a "short-timer."

Often in life we seem to feel as if we are "short-timers"; thus, we attempt to fill each day with more than twenty-four hours. We act as if we have only a few moments to live. Our society has become "eat, drink, and be merry, for tomorrow we die." In reality, we have only as many minutes to live as God allows.

The flowers on a cactus are "short-timers"; they are here for a few hours, days at the most, and then are gone. They are colors of the rainbow—yellow, red, white, and purple, just to name a few. The bees know the cactus flower is a "short-timer," and they work in the pollen rapidly, knowing that in a day or so at the most the nectar will be gone.

The experiences of life are often "short-timers," only lasting a few minutes, hours, or days. Thank goodness some of the experiences are "short-timers" because we humans could not endure the results if the times were longer. For example, women who give birth to a newborn are very happy that the birthing is a "short-time" experience. It must be something for the women who give birth to twins, quads, or in one case, seven babies. How they endure this situation is beyond a male's imagination.

When I am on a long flight, my wish is that it would be a "short-timer." Once while flying to Melbourne, Australia, we traveled nine hours to Auckland, New Zealand, and then had another three hours to our destination. After four or five hours, my wish was for the flight to end. But knowing it would not end caused me to attempt to believe that it was only a few more hours before my destination would be reached. In this way I was and am able to accept the conditions under which my flight is taking place.

Unlike some of the things we experience on this earth, God is not a "short-timer." The Bible states (paraphrased from 2 Peter 3:8) that a day is as a thousand years in His sight. When we pray, we desire God to answer prayer as of yesterday, but He will answer in His own good timing. It may be at once or, on the other hand, it may be years because He has the total picture in mind. We, as human beings, can only see or understand with our limited vision or understanding.

It is good that God is not a "short-timer." A book, written several years ago, and titled *Your God Is Too Small*, suggests that our concept of God is too small. As this book encourages, my vision has had to be enlarged concerning God. Until now, my thinking has been limited to my human wisdom. But today my understanding is expanding. Now I see how God can listen to prayers from His children all over the world—whether they speak different languages, have different colors of skin, or are in sad or excellent living conditions. I also see that God knows everything; His vision and knowledge are not limited as we humans are limited. He knows the very inner contents of our conscious and subconscious. Sometimes we humans believe we are able to hide our acts from God, but this is not so. All we do, think, and see He knows.

Often in my thinking, thoughts come to me that are improper, and I wonder, *Where in the world did that come from?* It came from the depths of my subconscious. When this occurs, I am pleased that with the assistance of God through Jesus Christ, my thought processes are "short-timers." In my conscious mind with the help of Scripture, unwanted thoughts can be erased. Satan has no chance against Scripture when we are invoking the name of Jesus Christ.

Is your life built on "short-timers"? I hope not.

When the Saints Go Marching In

DO YOU EVER think of what will happen to you when you die? It is my considered opinion that most humans think about this idea sometime in their lives. There are those souls who say they do not believe in God. But according to what polls have found here in the USA, 90 percent of the people in our nation believe in a God, and 70 percent say they pray each day. If these statistics are true, then most people think about what will happen to them when they die. Heaven and hell in some form must exist if these folks are telling us the truth.

The Bible discusses the facts of heaven and hell in strong terms. Heaven or paradise is the place prepared for those who believe in God and in Jesus Christ as He lived, died, and rose again on this earth. Hell is described in terms such as a place of eternal damnation, a lake of fire, and a never-ending burning of the human. Such descriptions in the Bible make most folks desire to be in heaven.

When Jesus Christ was dying on the cross, He told the repentant thief beside Him, "Today you will be with me in paradise." *Paradise* is a Persian word describing a beautiful garden where the pleasures of living are beyond the average person's expectations.

The Muslim concept of paradise is green grass; plenty of clean, fresh water; and seventy virgins. For this, today we have people willing to blow themselves up. If they die as martyrs, then the Koran assures them of going to paradise immediately.

It is the considered belief in the Christian faith that when you die, that is the end of human existence, and immediately after we leave this earth, after we draw our last breath, at once we are in the presence of God.

Depending on what branch of Judaism is espoused, some believe in an afterlife, and others do not. This is why the Jewish people do their good deeds on earth. To some degree, the Muslims do the same thing. They give at least two percent of their income to the poor.

Mankind looks into the skies and wonders what power brought this universe about. As far back as history is recorded, we humans have wondered about the cause of the being of this planet. Thinking people believe some power brought about what we see as the earth. They then wonder when human life ends once the body dies. People think that the cause which produced us could not have dropped us in a hole and said, "That is it."

We see the cycle of seasons. We see the planting of grain that produces something quite different from the item planted in the ground. Our sense of a greater power is evident in the coming together of the sperm and egg from which is produced a human, an animal of some species, a bird, or a reptile. Such observations make us believe that a greater power than man, which some of us call "God," produces all this.

So if the planting of a kernel of grain produces wheat, oats, corn, or soybeans, why then does this same power not cause mankind to continue after his body expires on this earth? True, we know of only a few people recorded to have been resurrected. These people have all been written about in the Bible; no scientific journal has seen the evidence of such action. We struggle with the record in the Bible and the scientific evidence that we do not have. Humankind longs for proof that resurrection takes place.

When the Saints Go Marching In

The early Egyptians believed that the soul returned to the body. As such, they went to great lengths to preserve the body, embalming it with great care. We see evidence of this procedure even in our time because these bodies are found mummified.

In China thousands of terra-cotta soldiers are all lined up to protect the monarch, who has been buried with such rituals. All his furniture, chariots, and clothes have been buried with these artifacts. Some sense of immortality existed in Chinese thinking many, many years ago.

Mankind has believed in a place for the good people and one for the bad. This is a common belief in all religions. What do you believe takes place when you die?

Resurrection

MANKIND DREAMS OF an afterlife but cannot decide what it will be.

The Muslims picture paradise as a place of great streams of running water, green grass in abundance, all the food you want to eat, and a great many beautiful women (all virgins).

The Jewish belief is only of the Messiah coming to this world. They believe that when He comes, everything will be beautiful. The Jewish nation will be established in the homeland. Wars of all types will cease; peace will be over the whole world. There is no concept of an afterlife as such. It is all tied with this earth.

In the time of Jesus, the Pharisees believed in a resurrection, and the Sadducees did not. Consequently, the Sadducees were in good with the Roman government. They curried favor with the Senate. The Pharisees wanted nothing to do with the Romans. They just put up with the Roman government because peace and stability came with their rule. Pharisees believed mankind would be judged in the last judgment according to the good deeds they had done on this earth. To them the resurrection was real.

The Hindus believe the afterlife is one continuous round of reincarnation. In this life you are a human being; in the next one you may be a monkey or a cow or any kind of animal or another human being. The human has the job of making sure his or her karma is proper so that he or she comes out the best possible way in the next life.

Christians believe that they will live for eternity in the presence of God—a God who is love, not hate; a Father who is more than the love of a human father. Christ told the thief beside Him on the cross, "Today you will be with me in Paradise." The word *Paradise* is a Persian idea. This concept is of a walled area with all the beauty to be found in a natural setting. Here mankind will live in the presence of God forever with fellow believers. No death, pain, or sorrow will be present. There will be complete joy and love beyond human understanding.

According to Scripture, the resurrection will come after the last judgment, when the good people and the evil people will be separated from each other forever. The Scripture speaks of a great canyon fixed between the good people and the evil ones. It will be impossible for the evil to cross over into the area of the good people, and this is all final. There is no second chance.

In the first century when the apostle Paul was asked to picture this soon after the death of Christ, he took a common example and used it to illustrate what will occur in the end of time. Paul states it like this: "You plant a grain of wheat in the soil. It dies. The following spring, after the rains come, the grain of wheat changes from a dead looking seed, to a thriving plant. It springs forth very different from the dead wheat seed planted by the farmer in the fall. This is similar to what happens in the Resurrection."

Our bodies die. Our souls go to be with God. And in the great judgment, the good shall come forth as completely new individuals, not with human bodies but with spiritual bodies. We shall be known as we were known while on this earth, but without any of the earthly limitations. Spiritual and physical limitations will be no more. We shall be like Christ. After His resurrection, He appeared as He wished and where He wished, even through closed doors.

Christians look forward to the resurrection and paradise that Jesus Christ spoke of the day He hung on the cross. The resurrection for the Christian means being released from the limitations we now have and living in the presence of all that is good and perfect.

The resurrection is a *wow* time!

Satan

DO YOU BELIEVE in Satan? There are scholars who claim he is only a figment of our imaginations. Do you agree? Sorry, but I believe he exists in many forms, and that all those forms are to catch the followers of God when they least expect it. I am one of those people.

Often wrong and harmful thoughts come to my mind when I least expect them. Then it occurs to me, *Where did that come from?* Has this ever happened to you? These thoughts are really harmful to my spiritual life. Dr. Freud would have said that these thoughts are from years of living and came from my unconscious. Maybe, but how did they get there to begin with?

Wrong or sinful thoughts coming unexpectedly in our minds is one of the things that convince me of the person of Satan.

Another way Satan attacks men of faith is with the current plague of beautiful women on the TV and Internet, where we are presented with hardly clad women selling every product on the market. All I need to do to have sexual pictures flood my computer screen is to type "sex," and an abundance of material rushes before my eyes. Sometimes I do not even need to do that, and it jumps out at me. Our TV and Internet sell on the flesh and bodies of beautiful women. Satan has been able to make a wedge into the sales market by using beautiful women's bodies. The sight of a female body arouses men. The subtle message is this: purchase this product, and you will have the female.

Now this approach is intended to catch the attention of men, but it also is made alluring to women. These things say to women "Act and dress like this, and your man or men will desire you as a sexual object." The subtle message is this: purchase this product, and you will be as beautiful as the female you see on the screen.

Satan has his agents working all the time to overcome the sense of value that God placed on the human form He created. It is a battle between God and Satan for the souls and bodies of the top creation by God. Satan delights in capturing one human soul and thus turning one made in the image and likeness of God into his product. Just imagine how he must laugh each time one of us humans falls for his "apple" message. Can't you hear him saying, "Got another one, God; You don't have them all."

Eve was not the only human being who believed the lie of Satan. Yes, we do know the difference between good and evil, but what a price we are paying for the apple. Venereal disease is rampant all over the world, killing millions of people and leaving millions of children orphans. The medical costs are eating up the financial wealth of the world as we battle the results of the satanic call.

Forty-six million babies have been killed in abortions because of the message of Satan. Folks go on enjoying sexual pleasure and then wonder why they feel guilty and unclean. They have believed in the lies of Satan. Sexual pleasure is a gift from God within the proper channels—that is, between one man and one woman in monogamy, not in polygamy, as practiced in our world culture today.

Satan is present in unconscious forms presented by the programs we see on TV. Regular soap operas that appear five days a week on TV flood the homes of millions of people and are viewed by females and retired fools who watch TV as daily entertainment. This "stuff" is plain "junk" and a product of evil minds who write for these programs. They do not care what they present, and Satan does his work through these people.

We see Satan at work in the growth of the gambling industry. We may have taken the land of the Native American tribes, but they are taking the money of the white folks with the casinos each and every tribe has on their properties. This is not true of only one state but of most of the states. An exception to this is the Navajo Nation. They have ruled out casinos because they see what is happening to other Native Americans where the casinos are present.

Many states now rake in large sums of money by the taxes exacted from the results of the casinos. The success of their casinos has made it possible for the tribes to do many projects not possible before; underneath, Satan is laughing because he has won with evil over good.

And it is not just gambling that shows Satan at work; betting is also prevalent. Today on this computer, I could gamble any amount of money desired by placing a bet over the Internet.

Satan goes on in his conquest of humankind. Last evening on the news, a story was run about the way men and some women are all tied up on certain football programs. These men act in foolish ways and are rude and sometimes very nasty toward their wives and families because of their addiction to the game. Here Satan wins again, this time over the good of the family. The family is a creation of God, started at the very beginning of the history of humankind.

Any way Satan can tear down the fabric of humankind and families satisfies his need to spit in the face of God.

Satan, may he rot in hell.

Why Are You on This Earth?

THAT'S A GOOD question: why are you on this earth? The Westminster Confession states, "Man's chief end is to glorify God and to enjoy him forever."

I ask, "How do you glorify God and enjoy him forever?" Learned theologians wrote this statement of faith many centuries ago. Religious divines have struggled with this statement over many generations. What does it mean to "glorify God"? How do you, a human being, enjoy Him forever? Allow me to attempt an answer.

To begin with, how do you glorify God? Is it by remembering you were created by His power? Genesis 1 states that God said, "Let us make man in our image, after our likeness" (v. 26). God also said, after looking over His creation (including man), "It is very good." So do we glorify God by admitting He created us?

We didn't just happen. Each time I see a new baby and the perfection that baby goes through in nine months, I am driven back to the fact that God, a divine presence, has a strong hand in the creative process. The delicate structure of the human body could have taken place only under the hand of God. We humans can produce amazing things, but nothing thus far can compare to the development of the human body and its various systems. My limited knowledge of the workings of the human mind compels me to sincerely believe God did the construction.

When I delve into the conscious and the unconscious, or the subconscious, what comes out in me, which I do not understand, overcomes my simple mind. As I study my conscious and unconscious, the material which surfaces from where I cannot tell is amazing, puzzling, and sometimes downright disturbing. I will often say, "Where did that come from? How did it get there?" The storehouse of material that comes to the surface is unbelievable. Sometimes I wish I could extinguish it, as with a fire hose in a house fire.

On the other hand, is glorifying God best shown when I love my neighbor as I love myself? This is impossible within our human abilities. We, on our own, cannot love our neighbor as we love ourselves. To top this off, we are commanded by Jesus Christ to love God first, and then the other is to follow. Some power that is greater than we are must cause this process to take place. Herein we see the Holy Spirit, the part of God that makes His home in each believer.

I ask again, why are you on this earth? I think the divines are right: "to glorify God and enjoy him forever," but what is a simple answer to this equation?

Well, one way to glorify God is to take care of my neighbor, no matter who he or she is. This could include things like feeding, clothing, housing, educating, and medicating. Jesus shared the good news; that is, man is a child of God and, as such, is to be loved even when unlovable.

Jesus told a Jewish scholar and member of the ruling religious body these words, "For God so loved the world that he gave his one and only Son, that whoever believes in him shall not perish but have eternal life. For God did not send his Son into the world to condemn the world, but to save the world through him" (John 3:16–17). Did God expect His Son to bring about the glorification of the Father? Apparently it was through the Son that mankind would glorify God. Mankind, by believing what the Son taught about God, would glorify Him. Yet all the time the New Testament points to Jesus Christ. The Holy Spirit directs the attention of the believer to Jesus Christ. So is this the method by which the human being glorifies God, by following the teachings of Jesus Christ?

Jesus Christ, speaking to His followers after His resurrection, stated, "I will send you the Comforter, even the Holy Spirit." God thus gives us the power to glorify Him by sending the Holy Spirit to live in the life of each and every believer. In this manner we are given the power to glorify God. As humans we do not possess this power. It is by the gift of God that we are given the power to glorify Him—we are given the power through the Holy Spirit, which is given to us upon our commitment to Jesus Christ.

If that is how we glorify God, how then do we enjoy God forever?

As I viewed the evening sunset, seeing the magic with which the western sky was painted in vivid colors, it was my privilege to enjoy God.

Each morning when I witness the rising of the sun in the eastern sky with its colors splashed over the horizon, I enjoy God.

When a rainbow appears high in the heavens and a rainstorm has preceded it, enjoyment of God is evident in my eyes.

When the dry desert springs to life, and flowers, which have appeared dead, jump to life, then God is enjoyed more fully in my human imagination.

Each time a mother quail runs across the road with her family of little ones, no larger than a silver dollar, the enjoyment of God gives me pleasure beyond imagination.

The smell of fresh rain upon our parched desert gives me exceeding pleasure.

The taste of a fresh peach on my tongue brings out the glory of God and the enjoyment of His power in creation.

Hearing music, which transports me into heavenly places, allows me to experience the enjoyment of God as He gives to mankind the ability to bring all the sounds into an experience beyond comprehension.

When I touch the soft skin of a newborn baby, the way God meant mankind to be rushes in upon me. It seems as if God has chosen to share a bit of Himself in that moment of touch.

When I hear of people being rescued from the results of their sin and accepting Jesus and all He did to save them, the joy of God comes to me fully.

As you read above, my ability to articulate what I mean by glorifying God is, at best, limited. But when the picture of enjoying God registers in my brain, I am more able to say what is coming from all five of my senses.

The Westminster confession divines were correct. Our chief end as human beings "is to glorify God and enjoy him forever."

Humility

THE WORD *HUMBLE* does not fit into the vocabulary of most Americans. We pride ourselves on being strong and able to go it alone; we do not need another person to help us. Yet those of us who claim to be Christians, whatever that may mean, are called upon to treat others as we wish to be treated. This concept is commonly called the Golden Rule.

Christ, after whom the word *Christian* originated, taught, "Thou shalt love the Lord thy God with all thy heart, soul, mind and strength, and thy neighbor as thyself." To care for another person is probably the most difficult task an individual has. To see that another person has what I have or, better yet, calls up the utmost strength is quite a challenge. On our own, we are incapable of doing this.

It is difficult for most of us even to think positive thoughts about our neighbors. We come into this world with a negative attitude. From the moment we take our first breath, our thinking is negative. We want our mother to pay attention only to our needs. We are selfish from the word *go*. Humility is not of our original making. If we do not get our way, there will be such a cry as one has never heard. From the word *go*, we expect to have the first and only place in the life of our mother. She has to give up all others to satisfy us.

If you think about it, to survive the baby has to take the first place in every thought of the chief caregiver. Probably this has to be. The mother lays her very life on the line to bring the child into the world. Even in this advanced medical age here in the United States, one out of every one thousand women dies in child birth. In the time of Abraham Lincoln, death from childbirth was a very common thing, and women entered into pregnancy with fear and trembling. A woman never knew if her life would be forfeited from the moment she conceived. Medical care was crude at best and often not available at all. This was especially true of the women living in the backcountry. They were without any care at all or, at best, had a midwife. The mother had to be a very humble person to lay her life on the line for the little one in her womb.

Humility seems to have been bred into women from the very first. In Old Testament times, women were often in despair because they could not conceive a child. Every woman wanted a son first and foremost. After she was able to have her husband's seed planted in her womb and it turned out to be a male, she felt life was complete.

Humility just seems to be part of the makeup of a female, even in the animal kingdom. The female animal will go to many lengths to become pregnant. Once that has occurred, she then goes about her business, feeding the little being inside her body.

When it comes to our dealing with other human beings, we often place ourselves in the position of "eating humble pie." This happened to me in the recent week. I did not think through what would take place when I made a certain statement. This, in turn, caused me much anguish. This lack of thinking through the statement before I made it caused me a great amount of concern until I had made lip restitution. I had to "eat humble pie," going to two people and making apologies for my words. It was necessary for me to humble myself to total strangers. I hope this experience will cause me to think long and hard before making a statement, even if it is honest; that is not correct on my part or before such an act of the tongue takes place again.

Whether my act of restitution will be accepted is yet to be seen. I was sincere in making the apology; there was no faking it. Actions that follow will indicate if my "eating humble pie" really was accepted by the people involved. Only time will tell.

LaVergne, TN USA
05 August 2010
192270LV00004B/5/P